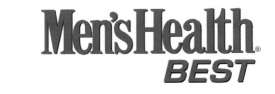

SPORTS INJURIES
HANDBOOK

Men's Health® BEST

SPORTS INJURIES HANDBOOK

SECRETS FROM *MEN'S HEALTH* MAGAZINE

Edited by **Joe Kita**, *Men's Health* magazine

RODALE

This edition first published in 2005 by
Rodale International Ltd
7–10 Chandos Street
London
W1G 9AD
www.rodalebooks.co.uk

"Men's Health®" is a registered trademark of Rodale Inc.

Cover photograph by Pablo Arroyo; back cover photograph by Getty Images.

Interior Photographs
Comstock: 23; Eyewire: 30, 39, 53; John Hamel/Rodale Image Library: 6, 7, 79, 90; Image Source: 10; Michael Mazzeo: 18, 19, 20, 21, 22, 31, 32, 33, 34, 35, 36, 37, 38, 45, 46 ,47, 48, 49, 50, 51, 52, 59, 60, 61, 62, 63, 64, 65, 66, 91, 92, 93, 94; Photodisc: 11; Primal Pictures: 12, 16, 24, 29, 40, 43, 54, 57, 68, 70, 71, 72, 73, 74, 75, 76, 77, 78, 80, 81, 83, 85, 86, 88; Rodale Image Library: 17; Sally Ullman/Rodale Image: 67; Kurt Wilson/Rodale Image Library: 7.

Printed and bound in China.
3 5 7 9 8 6 4

A CIP catalogue record for this book is available from the British Library.

ISBN 978-1-4050-7765-1

Notice
The information in this book is meant to supplement, not replace, proper exercise training. All forms of exercise pose some inherent risks. The editors and publisher advise readers to take full responsibility for their safety and know their limits. Before practising the exercises in this book, be sure that your equipment is well maintained, and do not take risks beyond your level of experience, aptitude, training and fitness.

The exercise and dietary programmes in this book are not intended as a substitute for any exercise routine or dietary regime that may have been prescribed by your doctor. As with all exercise and dietary programmes, you should get your doctor's approval before beginning.

Visit us on the Web at *www.menshealth.co.uk*

LIVE YOUR WHOLE LIFE™

We inspire and enable people to improve their lives and the world around them

CONTENTS

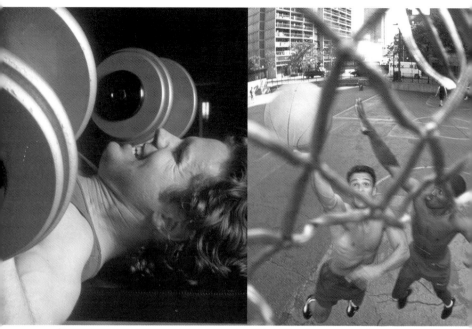

Get back in the game: rebounding from a sports injury takes a little patience and a lot of know-how.

INTRODUCTION

What was *that*? How many times have you been running, lifting or playing football when you've heard the thing you dread? The pop. The crunch. The sensation of something tearing in your knee, shoulder or ankle. Before the pain arrives, there's the familiar dread. Then, as you ice the swollen joint, you wonder: how did this happen? What will the doctor say? How can I prevent this from happening in the future?

This book answers all of those questions and offers workout programmes – designed by professionals – to help you rebuild strength and flexibility after any injury. It also includes expert medical and exercise advice that will help you *safely* get back to your pre-injury fitness level without stressing your healing bones, joints and muscles. If you aren't hurt now, use the workouts and prevention tips in each section to make a pre-emptive strike against future sports injuries.

Are Your Workouts to Blame?

It's not just the collision on the field or a bad landing after a jump

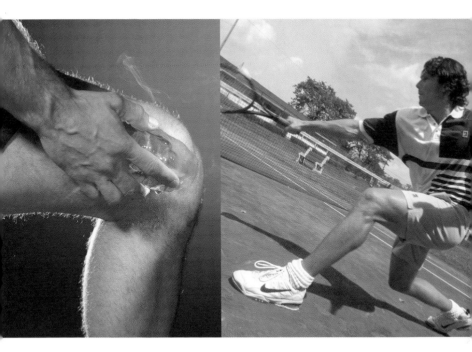

that can have you limping to the sidelines. Failing to balance your workouts or working some muscles too much while ignoring others can leave you vulnerable to injuries.

Over-training is the surest way to end up in a doctor's surgery because you're beating down your muscles with each gruelling session. Tired muscles fatigue the tendons that hold the muscles to your bones. The tendons swell and if you work out through the pain, your tendons can begin to scar – nagging aches during workouts can be a sign that you're overworking the muscles and tendons in your body. Eventually, you'll pay for pushing your body too hard.

One method to prevent over-training is to follow the 10 per cent rule. Don't increase the distance you run, the speed of your runs or the weight that you lift by more than 10 per cent per week. This gives your tendons, muscles and bones a chance to adapt to each new workload.

How to Use This Book

Each section in this book focuses on the most common sports-related injuries that affect every part of the body, from the feet to the hands, the back to the shoulders. You'll learn how the injury feels, how it probably happened, how to treat the injury and how to prevent such an injury

TREATING INJURIES WITH RICE

Pain and swelling is the body's way of telling you that something has gone wrong. You can help your body heal and keep things from getting worse, if you know what to do. The best system for dealing with almost every sports injury is the **RICE** method. RICE stands for **R**est, **I**ce, **C**ompression and **E**levation.

What does *rest* mean? Generally, it means stopping doing what you were doing when you got injured. If you've got an ankle that's black and blue and swelling up like a basketball, then don't walk on it. Protect it with crutches or a walking stick. If it's just a minor sprain, you'll want to move it a little, to put some weight on it to see how it feels. In general, your body will 'splint' an injury, making it as immobile as it's supposed to be. Try to move any joint that's injured. If you can't move it, or if the pain is unbearable, then your body is telling you to leave it alone and hurry to the doctor.

Ice should be applied to the swelling for twenty minutes every four to six hours for the first day or two. Keep applying ice until the pain and swelling go down. Protect your skin from frostbite by wrapping the ice in a towel.

Compression means pressure is applied to keep the swelling down, usually using tape or a bandage. In some cases, it's fairly easy to apply pressure to the area around the injury. For example if you've sprained your ankle, don't remove your shoe right away. The compression provided by your shoe will help keep the swelling down until you can locate an ice pack.

Keeping the injured body part *elevated* above your heart will help reduce pain and swelling by keeping the fluids from building up at the site of your injury.

---

from recurring. From there, you can turn to the expert-designed workouts, where you'll find exercises to help you rehabilitate existing injuries and strengthen the body part so you don't get injured again.

Warm Up to Your Workout

Never go full-speed in your workout until you've warmed up and broken into a light sweat. This indicates that your core body temperature is high enough to make your tendons and ligaments pliable. It also ensures that your cartilage – and the bones it protects – is well lubricated. Generally speaking, stretching is a good way to improve flexibility; however, stretching just before a workout or sports activity is not necessarily an effective way to prevent injury. Instead, warm up with five to ten minutes of low-impact cardiovascular exercise, such as jogging or cycling, before a game or weight-training session. Then, stretch after you warm up and after the game – when your muscles and tendons are more pliable.

A Balanced Programme

All workout programmes need to be balanced. This is especially important after you've suffered a sports-related injury, and can mean the difference between a swift and safe return to play or a prolonged layoff.

Flip through each section to determine which workouts best target the bones, muscles and joints affected by your injury. Then, read through the workout introductions and exercise descriptions to see if the demands of the programme suit your fitness level. In some instances, the workout included in a section may contain exercises that are not appropriate for you if you are recovering from certain injuries.

Pay close attention to the flexibility and strengthening exercises recommended for each injury – in many cases, you'll be referred to specific preventative exercises or to complete workout programmes. If you have additional concerns about physical limitations as they may relate to your injury, consult your doctor before beginning any of the workout programmes in this book.

Stay Injury-Free

Perform your workout every other day, three times a week, for four to six weeks. Warm up for each weight-training session with 5 to 10 minutes of low-impact cardiovascular exercise. Then, work through the flexibility and strength-training exercises in the order they appear. Rest for 30 seconds to a minute between exercise sets and when moving from one exercise to the next. When you're working with heavier weights and lower reps, you may need longer rest periods. On the days you aren't lifting, do up to 45 minutes of low-impact aerobic exercise.

As you work out, keep in mind that all sets, reps and weights are suggested benchmarks that you may need to work up to. Although all the exercises are safe, you should *always* listen to your body when weight-training and never lift a weight or hold a stretch to the point of pain.

Handling the Pain

For many minor injuries, over-the-counter pain medications, such as ibuprofen or paracetamol, will help relieve pain. Also use RICE (see page 8) to control pain and swelling.

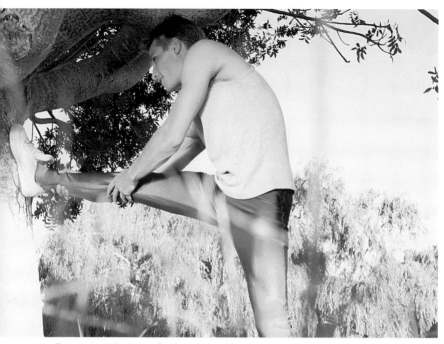

Recovery is a balancing act: find the right mix of flexibility and strength training, and learn the difference between pushing yourself and pushing yourself too hard. Over-training will put you back on the bench.

Getting Back in the Game

The first rule of rehabilitation is to take it easy. Don't rush it. This is especially true if your injury required surgery to repair torn ligaments and tendons. Your rehab goals should be:

1. Restore your range of motion in the injured joint. You can't play on it if you can't move it.
2. Restore your flexibility by stretching every day to speed healing and relieve pain.
3. Restore your strength and endurance by gradually increasing the demands of your workout programme. Use cross-training to maintain your overall fitness level and sport-specific exercises to prepare your body for a return to your activity.
4. Restore your sense of balance and co-ordination. Exercises such as balancing on one foot with your eyes closed help to remind your brain how to sense and move a newly healed leg.

The ultimate goal, of course, is to return to your game at your pre-injury fitness level. This could take a few days or several months, depending on how severe your injury is.

Foot, Ankle and Lower-Leg Injuries

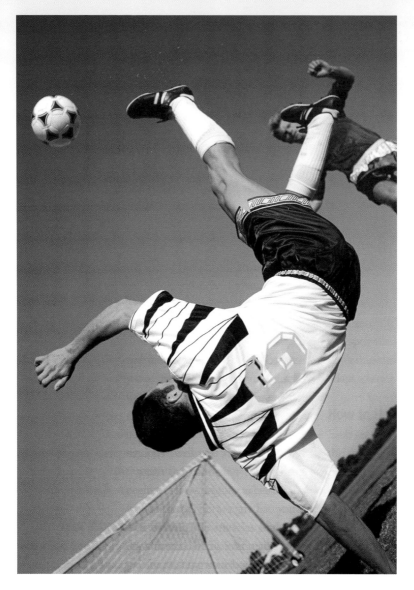

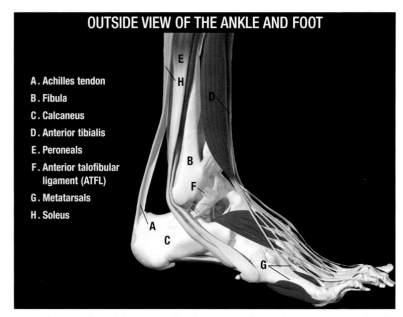

OUTSIDE VIEW OF THE ANKLE AND FOOT

A. Achilles tendon
B. Fibula
C. Calcaneus
D. Anterior tibialis
E. Peroneals
F. Anterior talofibular
   ligament (ATFL)
G. Metatarsals
H. Soleus

Your feet and ankles were built to comfortably carry your body weight all day long, and most of the time they do an admirable job. Unfortunately, pounding the pavement on long runs or making sudden moves on the court can cause strains or stress fractures that will keep you off your feet for weeks or even months. Most people don't take the time to stretch and warm up these muscles and tendons properly before every workout and game. Others don't bother to buy shoes that fit. If this sounds like you, you may have foot complications in your future. Here's a breakdown of the most common sports-related foot, ankle and lower-leg injuries.

PULLED OR TORN ACHILLES

How it feels

You hear a pop in the cord-like Achilles tendon that runs along the back of your ankle followed by pain and swelling. In some cases, these signs of injury may appear the day after a workout. It's difficult to walk and you may not be able to push up onto your toes without pain.

How it happened

You took off at a sudden sprint or went running uphill. Your calf muscles may be tight and inflexible.

How to treat it

Use RICE (see page 8) to reduce the pain and swelling. You may need crutches or heel lifts to keep pressure off your tendon while it heals. Be sure to get lifts in both shoes or you'll throw your back out. If the Achilles tendon is completely torn, you will need surgery.

How to prevent it

Even if you don't exercise daily, work on improving the flexibility of your calf muscles and the Achilles tendon with the stretches on pages 18–19.

HEEL PAIN

How it feels

Heel pain, also known as plantar fasciitis, causes pain on the bottom of the foot at or near the heel and radiating up into the arch of the foot. The pain may be worse first thing in the morning and during long runs.

How it happened

The plantar fascia tendon that runs along the bottom of your foot has tightened because you've been running without stretching properly or because your arches are very high.

What a doctor will tell you

Stretching exercises that lengthen the achilles tendon and plantar fascia (see pages 18–19) will make the tendon more flexible over time. If the pain is very bad, you may want to try using heel inserts or even a cortisone injection.

How to prevent it

Stretch. Make sure your shoes fit properly and are replaced regularly, about every 650 to 800 kilometres (400 to 500 miles).

SPRAINED ANKLE

How it feels

You may hear a pop at the time of the injury, followed by pain, swelling or bruising around your ankle.

How it happened

You may have torn one or all of the ligaments that help hold the outside of the ankle joint together.

How to treat it

Use RICE to control the swelling. You'll also want to try to move your ankle a bit. Increasing blood circulation around the injury speeds the healing process and relieves pain. Rotate the ankle gently to start this process. If you can't move it or if you experience extreme pain when you try, the bones could be broken and it's time to go to hospital. If not, use RICE for a few days along with medication. Use an ankle brace to support the ankle while the torn ligaments heal.

FALLEN ARCHES AND METATARSALGIA

Fallen arches (Pes Planus) can occur over time or if your arches have never fully developed. Flat feet – the opposite of a high arch – may contribute to pain around the inside of the ankle extending to the foot. Running too far on flat feet will irritate the posterior tibialis tendon and cause pain and swelling. Use RICE to relieve the pain and invest in shoe inserts, called orthotics, to prevent further injury.

When the pain is located on the balls of your feet, instead of the arch, your doctor may call this metatarsalgia. It means the bones in your feet hurt because you've been abusing them. This problem often results from wearing running shoes that are too tight or simply having feet with an abnormally high arch. If you have a high arch, you may need shoe supports for your feet.

How to prevent it

Don't exercise on uneven, slippery surfaces and avoid training on grassy, rocky or sandy terrain. Use an ankle brace when you work out.

ANKLE FRACTURE

How it feels

If you hear crunching sounds coming from your ankle, it may be the first hint that you're suffering from more than just a sprain. That sound will be followed by searing pain, swelling and bleeding under the skin. You will be unable to stand.

How it happened

The tibia and fibula, the two bones that make up your shins, have broken at the point where they join the foot. Because there are so many different types of breaks, a doctor should make the diagnosis. Depending on the severity of the fracture, you'll be sidelined for anywhere from six weeks to three months.

How to treat it

First, you'll need an X-ray, then a cast and crutches, a splint or a walking frame.. You may even need surgery.

How to prevent it

The only thing you can do is watch your step when you are playing.

STRESS FRACTURES OF THE FOOT

How it feels

There is swelling and aching pain in the bones of your feet, particularly in the metatarsals – the long bones that run through the middle of the foot and behind each toe. The pain can seem generalized, like tendonitis, or centred on one specific spot.

How it happened

Hairline breaks in the foot bones are an overuse injury often caused by running too far, running too fast and too often, or not regularly replacing your running shoes. When you quickly increase the distance you run, or run on a hard terrain, the bones in your feet absorb more impact and gradually break down from too much wear. Ultimately, you get stress fractures.

How to treat it

This type of injury doesn't always show up on an X-ray. You can get an MRI test – which provides computer-generated images of the body – or treat it as a stress fracture until the pain goes away. Use RICE to control the pain and swelling. Emphasize *rest* to let the bones repair themselves. When it's time to return to running, increase your distance slowly – 10 per cent per week – to prevent a recurrence. Also, try to run on soft surfaces, such as a smooth dirt track or even grass.

How to prevent it

Wear athletic shoes with good shock-absorption. Steadily build up the distance you jog and the amount of time you work out.

PERONEAL TENDONITIS

How it feels

You have pain and swelling around your ankle along the peroneal tendons. You may have heard a pop when the injury happened.

How it happened

You overused the outside of your ankle or turned your ankle inwards. This has torn or stretched the tendon on the outside of the ankle.

· HIGH ANKLE SPRAIN

A high ankle sprain is like an ordinary sprain except that you landed on your toes and rolled the foot all the way over. This separates the two shinbones (tibia and fibula) and sprains the ligaments in between them. It is difficult to walk and there is pain up the shinbone. The recovery takes much longer than a sprained ankle and often requires prolonged immobilization.

INSIDE VIEW OF THE CALF, ANKLE AND FOOT

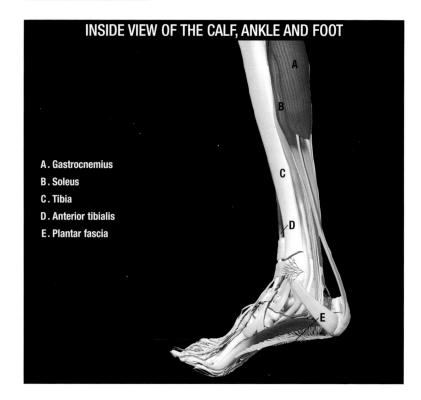

A. Gastrocnemius
B. Soleus
C. Tibia
D. Anterior tibialis
E. Plantar fascia

How to treat it

Use RICE to relieve swelling. Before you work out, be sure to warm up your ankles with pain-free range-of-motion exercises (see pages 19–22) to preserve flexibility and mobility of your ankle joints. You may need physiotherapy to strengthen the muscles surrounding your ankle. Temporary bracing, to immobilize the tendon, can be helpful.

How to prevent it

Stretch and strengthen your ankle joints and muscles using the exercises on pages 18–22.

SHIN SPLINTS
How it feels

The term *shin splints* describes pain over the front of the lower leg and is associated with inflammation of the tissue that covers the tibia (shinbone). You will feel sharp pain along the inside of your shins concentrated along the bone or in the muscles on the inside of the shinbone.

How it happened

This is an overuse injury to the bone or the muscles in your lower leg. Too much running on a hard surface with flat feet could be the culprit.

How to treat it

The location of the pain will tell you a lot about the type of injury. Pain on the tibia may indicate the beginnings of a stress fracture. If the pain is along the inside of the tibia, you are likely suffering from a shin splint. Pain and tightness in the meaty part of the shin just outside of the shinbone may be what's called compartment syndrome – swelling of the muscles on your shin that tense up when you run. Use RICE to control the pain and swelling. Decrease the intensity and frequency of your workouts to keep the situation from getting worse.

How to prevent it

Runners who over-pronate – tilt the ankle inwards and strike the ground with the inside of the foot – are susceptible to shin injuries. You can get orthotic pads for your shoes to help correct the angle of your foot strike.

CALF STRAIN

How it feels

You hear a loud pop and feel sudden pain in your calf. In some cases, you may feel just a twinge followed by pain, swelling and bruising.

How it happened

The muscles on the back of your leg were pushed further than they wanted to go. Sudden moves on the tennis court or on the football pitch can force the calf muscles to lengthen instantly. When they are unprepared for this, they tear.

How to treat it

Use RICE, non-steroidal pain medication and crutches if necessary.

How to prevent it

Warm up your whole leg with five to ten minutes of stationary cycling. Then, loosen up your muscles with the stretches on pages 18–19.

THE WET FOOTPRINT TEST

Wet the bottom of your foot; step onto a flat surface. Look at the footprint: if there's no arch, your feet roll too far inwards (over-pronate), which can lead to tendinitis. If the arch is high, your weight lands on the outside edge of your foot, making you susceptible to ankle sprains and stress fractures.

Normal   No Arch   High Arch

Foot, Ankle and Lower-Leg Workout

The swelling has gone down, the bruises have healed and you can finally ditch the crutches and the ankle brace. If you're ready to get off the sidelines – and stay off them – the following workout can help you safely re-develop strength and flexibility in the muscle groups of the foot, ankle and lower legs. Warm up with 5 to 10 minutes of low-impact aerobic exercise, then perform the strengthening and conditioning exercises in the order they appear below. As you work through the exercises, use the recommended sets, reps and weights as benchmarks – focus on performing each rep with perfect form to maximize strength gains and to minimize the risk of undue stress on your healing joints and muscles.

GASTROC STRETCH

Targets: Gastrocnemius, Plantor Fascia

Stand with your feet shoulder-width apart and place your hands on a wall in front of you. Extend your left leg behind you and slightly bend your right knee. Keeping your left leg straight and your heel on the ground, lean forwards until you first feel the stretch in the calf of your left leg. Hold for 5 deep breaths, or 20–30 seconds. Do 2 sets with each leg.

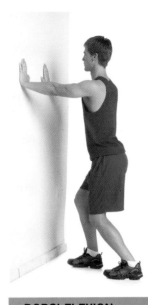

SOLEUS STRETCH

Targets: Soleus, Plantor Fascia

Stand with your feet shoulder-width apart and place your hands on a wall in front of you. With your right knee bent slightly, position your left leg behind you so the toe is in line with the heel of your right foot. Perform a partial squat by gently bending both knees until you feel a stretch in the lower calf of your left leg. Hold for 5 deep breaths, or 20–30 seconds. Do 2 sets with each leg.

DORSI FLEXION

Targets: Anterior Tibialis

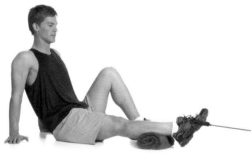

1. Sit on the floor and rest your lower calf on a towel. Secure one end of a piece of medium-resistance elastic exercise tubing to a bench or table and wrap the other end around the ball of your right foot.

2. Slowly pull the toes of your right foot towards you and hold 1–2 seconds. Rest, then repeat until you first feel fatigue in your right shin. Do 1 set to fatigue with each foot.

PLANTAR FLEXION

Targets: Gastrocnemius

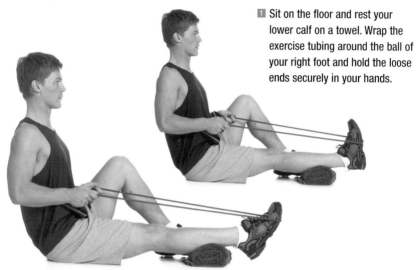

1️⃣ Sit on the floor and rest your lower calf on a towel. Wrap the exercise tubing around the ball of your right foot and hold the loose ends securely in your hands.

2️⃣ Point your right foot away from you and hold 1–2 seconds. Rest, then repeat until you first feel fatigue in your calf. Do 1 set to fatigue with each foot.

INVERSION

Targets: Anterior Tibialis, Posterior Tibialis

1️⃣ Sit on the floor and rest your lower calf on a towel. Secure one end of the exercise tubing to a bench or table and wrap the other end around the ball of your right foot.

2️⃣ Slowly turn your right foot inwards and hold 1–2 seconds. Rest, then repeat until you first feel fatigue along your right shin. Do 1 set to fatigue with each foot.

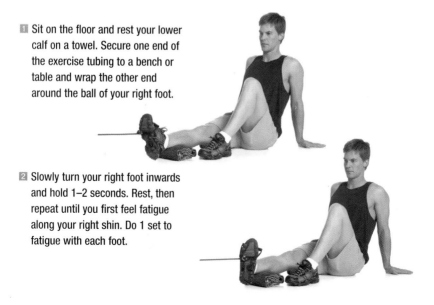

EVERSION

Targets: Peroneals

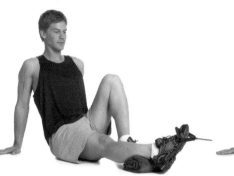

1. Sit on the floor and rest your lower calf on a towel. Secure one end of the tubing to a bench or table and wrap the other end around the ball of your right foot. Tilt your right foot slightly inwards.

2. Slowly turn your right foot outwards and hold 1–2 seconds. Rest, then repeat until you first feel fatigue along the outside of your right shin. Do 1 set to fatigue with each foot.

SITTING ALPHABET

Targets: Anterior Tibialis, Peroneals, Gastrocnemius, Posterior Tibialis

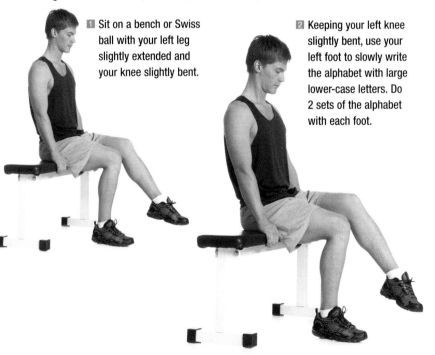

1. Sit on a bench or Swiss ball with your left leg slightly extended and your knee slightly bent.

2. Keeping your left knee slightly bent, use your left foot to slowly write the alphabet with large lower-case letters. Do 2 sets of the alphabet with each foot.

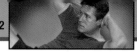

SINGLE LEG STANCE WITH OPPOSITE HIP CIRCLES

Targets: Anterior Tibialis, Peroneals, Gastrocnemius, Posterior Tibialis, Hip Flexor, Abductors, Buttocks, Hamstrings

1 Stand on your left leg and try to keep your balance. If you have an injury, practise on your non-injured leg first. If you have weight-bearing constraints on the injured ankle, consult your doctor.

2 With your hands on your hips, look straight ahead and extend your right foot in front of you.

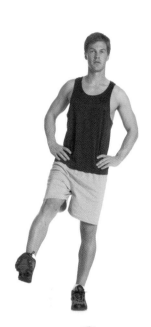

3 Extend your right leg to the side and slowly do a full hip circle.

4 Do 2 sets of 10 circles (5 clockwise and 5 counter-clockwise) with each leg.

Knee Conditions

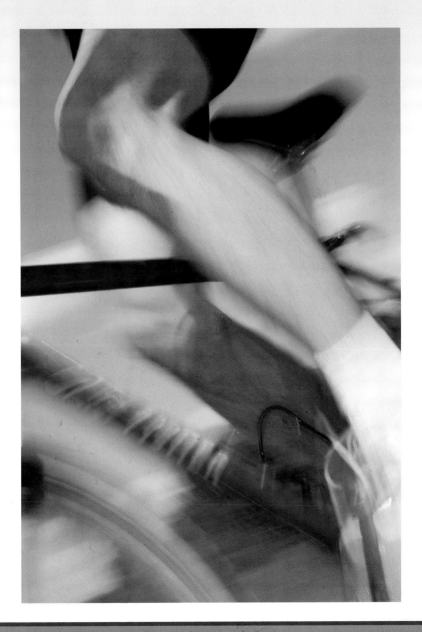

FRONT VIEW OF THE KNEE

A. Femur
B. Tibia
C. Patella
D. Fibula/fibular head
E. Medial meniscus
F. Patellar tendon
G. Lateral collateral ligament (LCL)
H. Iliotibial band
I. Vastus lateralis
J. Vastus medialis oblique (VMO)

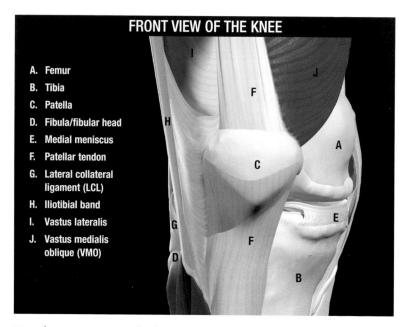

Your knee is a marvel of construction. One ligament on the outside (LCL) and one on the inside (MCL) hold your thigh bone to your shin bones. Two more ligaments (the ACL and PCL) cross inside the knee to keep the joint steady from front to back. In addition, cartilage inside the knee acts as a shock absorber. Keeping the muscles around your knees strong and supple can reduce your chances of suffering an injury that will leave you sidelined for the rest of the season.

ILIOTIBIAL BAND SYNDROME

How it feels

You feel a generalized pain on the outside of the knee. It's common amongst runners and cyclists. The pain gets worse when you run downhill or walk down stairs. By contrast, walking with stiff legs makes the pain go away.

How it happened

The iliotibial band (IT band) is a massive swathe of muscle and tendon that stretches from your pelvis to your knee. At the bottom of the femur, the IT band wraps over the outside of your knee bursa – a sack of fluid that protects the bone. If you run or cycle too far, your bursa swells and rubs against the bone.

How to treat it

Treating the injury with RICE (see page 8) will help reduce the pain and swelling. After that, do the stretches on pages 32–33 to increase the flexibility of the iliotibial band. Then, work on strengthening the outer muscles of the thigh with the exercises on pages 49–50.

How to prevent it

Most streets are cambered, meaning that their surface is uneven. Running on such surfaces can cause iliotibial band injuries. Where it is safe to do so, alternate running with and against traffic to compensate.

RUNNER'S KNEE
How it feels

Runner's knee causes throbbing pain behind the patella (kneecap). You'll feel it after (and sometimes during) a run, when you come up from a squat, while lunging or after you've been sitting for an extended period.

How it happened

Your kneecap travels up and down in a groove as you walk or run. If you run too frequently with poor form, your kneecap can slip off track a bit and rub away the protective cartilage behind it. This can be caused by flat feet, a muscle imbalance or over-training. The more tired the muscles in your knees are, the less capable they are of holding everything in place.

How to treat it

Ice the area around your knee to reduce the pain and then think about scaling back on the sports you play. Reducing your activity is important, because this condition can lead to chondromalacia, in which the cartilage is worn away by friction. Cross-train for a few weeks during the healing process.

How to prevent it

Avoid full squats, lunges and the leg extension machine at the gym. Increase your flexibility with the stretches on pages 32–33 and strengthen your leg muscles with the exercises on pages 33–34.

JUMPER'S KNEE
How it feels

Patellar tendinitis, more commonly referred to as jumper's knee, causes pain on the front of the knee below the kneecap while squatting, running, kneeling and jumping.

How it happened

Landing after a jump loads many times your body weight onto your knees and the tendons that hold the muscles to the bones. Over time, the patellar tendon that connects the kneecap to the shinbone becomes inflamed and causes swelling.

How to treat it

Use RICE to control the pain and swelling around your knee. Focus on developing strength in your thigh muscles with Partial Quadriceps Extensions (page 37) and Leg Raises (pages 33–34) to reduce the strain on the patellar tendon. You may want try using orthotics – special shoe inserts that can be used to correct pronation problems. You can also try a patellar band – a strip of elastic you wear beneath your kneecap to keep your patellar tendon braced, minimizing stress on your knee. With patellar tendinitis,

DISLOCATED KNEECAP

While your knee was twisting itself out of alignment, your kneecap may have popped out of its groove. You'll know if this has happened because the kneecap will look deformed and hurt like hell. If you can find a way to straighten your knee, it will sometimes pop back in. Even if it slides back into place on its own, see your doctor as soon as you can. Ice it and keep it straight.

you can usually play through some of the pain as long as it does not progressively worsen.

How to prevent it

Avoid full leg extension machines at the gym. Rather than developing muscle, you may irritate the tendons that support your knee and quad muscles. Instead, try modified exercises using leg press machines, such as the Leg Press with Ball Squeeze (page 35), to build more muscle and minimize stress on your knee.

MENISCAL CARTILAGE TEAR

How it feels

The injury itself may not be as painful as you would think. But over time, you will feel pain in and around your knee when going up stairs or hills, or when you do a full squat. You may even hear clicking in your knee joint as you move. Sometimes, your knee may seize up.

How it happened

While walking or running, you damaged one of the two rubbery pieces of cartilage inside your knee that keep your thighbone from rubbing directly against your shinbone. The cartilage can also be worn down with use or you may just twist your knee getting up from the floor.

How to treat it

Of the usual treatments, rest is the most important. The meniscus cannot heal without rest, and sometimes a minor tear can heal on its own. In other cases, you will need surgery to repair the damage. The Leg Raises on pages 33–34 can also help in the healing.

How to prevent it

Minimize squatting and twisting your knee joint. Maintain flexibility with the stretches on pages 32–33.

STRESS FRACTURE

How it feels

You will feel progressive, nagging pain in the kneecap or shinbone that gets worse during workouts.

How it happened

You have been over-training to the extent that the bones in your leg or knee have not been able to regenerate. Instead, they have been breaking down. As a result, you have the beginning of a hairline fracture in one of the bones of your knee.

How to treat it

Ice and pain medication can reduce the swelling and discomfort, but most importantly, stop training. Take at least a month away from training to let the bones heal. If the injury is serious, you may need physiotherapy to safely work the muscles around the fracture. In any case, you'll want to rebuild bone *and* muscle before you return to your sport.

How to prevent it

Increase training gradually to let the bone adapt to your running or weight-lifting programme.

TORN ACL

How it feels

First, you'll hear a pop or snap, like a rubber band breaking inside your leg. You may also feel your knee buckle and no longer support you. The knee will swell quickly as the tissue around the ligament bleeds into your knee joint – that's when the pain really intensifies.

How it happened

Your shinbone has been pulled or twisted away from the knee, and the anterior cruciate ligament (ACL), which holds the front of the knee together, has snapped under the pressure. In skiing, it's because the knee turned in one direction while the ski kept the rest of your leg planted somewhere else; or maybe you fell back on your skis and tried to recover your balance. In tennis or football, it probably occurred during a pivot or a sudden stop.

How to treat it

Don't walk on it. Use RICE and try to elevate the leg as quickly as possible to contain the swelling. If you are in excruciating pain, a doctor can drain blood and fluid from the knee using a syringe – a process known as aspiration – to help relieve pain and reduce swelling. Wear a brace that allows full range of motion but still supports your knee.

Surgery isn't always necessary; it depends on your age, activity level, the stability of your knee and the condition of any other structures in the knee that may also be damaged. Physiotherapy, however, is crucial. It will help you build strength in the muscles around the knee while it heals, and will improve your range of motion. Be careful not to push your knee beyond what is therapeutic.

A minor sprain needs at least four weeks to heal. A complete tear with reconstructive surgery will require four to six months of recovery time.

How to prevent it

Learn from an expert in your sport how to land from a jump and how to train the hamstring muscles to better alleviate a sudden load on the ACL. Such hamstring strengthening may help, but make sure to balance the workout by also training muscles on the front of the leg. Try to restore flexibility and strength in your knee with the stretches and exercises on pages 31–38.

TORN MCL

How it feels

A torn medial collateral ligament (MCL) causes a sharp pain on the inside of your knee.

How it happened

Any hit on the outer part of the knee may tear the MCL. Twisting your knee may also force it to buckle inwards, stretching the MCL.

How to treat it

Ice the area around the injury to reduce pain and swelling. Invest in a brace that will stabilize the knee for a couple of months while it heals. The brace should provide support while allowing full range of motion to speed healing. Physiotherapy will help strengthen the muscles around the injury and maintain flexibility. You probably won't need surgery unless it's a catastrophic tear. There are many degrees of tearing, from grade one (least severe) to grade three (most severe).

How to prevent it

If you know you may be hit on the outer part of the knee, wear a hinged brace to help absorb the shock and

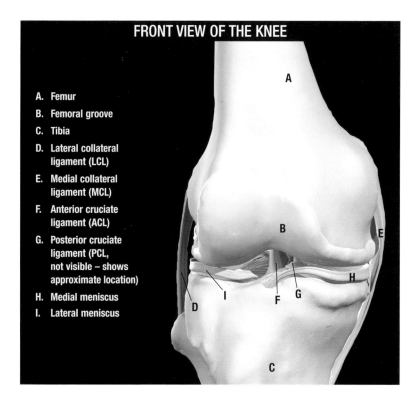

FRONT VIEW OF THE KNEE

A. Femur
B. Femoral groove
C. Tibia
D. Lateral collateral ligament (LCL)
E. Medial collateral ligament (MCL)
F. Anterior cruciate ligament (ACL)
G. Posterior cruciate ligament (PCL, not visible – shows approximate location)
H. Medial meniscus
I. Lateral meniscus

decrease the severity of the injury. Do the flexibility and strengthening exercises on pages 31–38.

TORN LCL
How it feels
It's the opposite of an MCL injury; in this case, the sharp pain is on the outside of the knee.

How it happened
This injury is rarer than other types of knee injuries. The most likely cause is stopping or starting sud-denly and your knee buckling out-wards. Perhaps you were tackled and your knee was forced outwards.

How to treat it
Treat with RICE and make an appointment to see your doctor – it's rare to have an injury to the lateral collateral ligament (LCL) alone. Any accident that takes out the LCL has probably torn other ligaments or car-tilage as well. Wear a brace and get some physiotherapy to strengthen the knee and maintain your ability

to move it properly. A torn LCL can keep you out of action anywhere from four to twelve weeks.

How to prevent it

Do the flexibility and strengthening exercises on pages 31–38.

SILENT PCL TEAR
How it feels

The primary symptoms are mild to moderate pain on the back of the knee. The pain will be manageable; your knee may feel slightly wobbly.

How it happened

You fell on your bent knee or it hit the dashboard of a car during a crash. The posterior cruciate ligament (PCL) can tear when something hits the front of the knee, forcing it backwards.

How to treat it

Pain is usually a good indicator of how serious an injury is – more pain usually means more severe tearing. This is not the case with a silent PCL tear. Even moderate pain on the back of the knee can be a signal of serious tearing that needs to be evaluated by a doctor. If left untreated, a torn PCL can contribute to arthritis later in life. You may need surgery to repair it, although many people heal without surgery. You'll miss anywhere from four to eight weeks of activity without surgery and from four to six months with it.

How to prevent it

Develop strength and flexibility in the muscles around your knees with the exercises on pages 31–38.

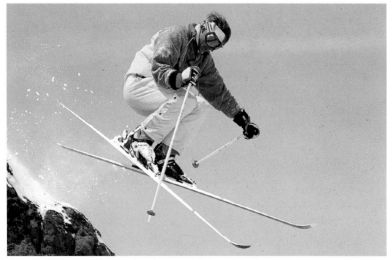

Strong, healthy knees will help you jump from great heights, and then land safely.

Knee Workout

Good form is critical when training the knee. Why? Because any strengthening exercise performed with improper technique can create muscular imbalance – the root of most sports-related injuries. After warming up with 5 to 10 minutes of low-impact aerobic exercise, ease into your workout with the flexibility moves and pay close attention to make sure you do each exercise with perfect form. If you experience any pain, decrease the range of motion until you can do the exercise without pain or discomfort. Then, gradually increase the range of motion until you can perform the move as described. The exercises that follow are designed to help correct common technique flaws that can aggravate underlying conditions or cause new injuries.

QUAD STRETCH
Targets: Quadriceps

Standing on your left leg, bend your right knee and grab your foot with your right hand. Without leaning forwards, flex your right knee and gently pull your leg back until you feel a stretch in your right quad. If you have a hard time keeping your balance, use a wall or chair for support. Hold for 4–5 deep breaths, or 20–30 seconds. Do 2 sets with each leg.

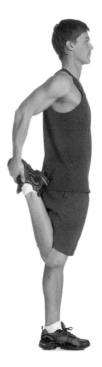

SEATED HAMSTRING STRETCH

Targets: Hamstrings

In a seated position, extend your right leg straight in front of you and pull your left leg towards your groin. Look straight ahead and slowly lean forwards until you feel a stretch in your right hamstring. Don't arch your back to get more of a stretch; keep your chest out and your back straight to avoid stress on your lower back. Hold for 4–5 deep breaths, or 20–30 seconds. Do 2 sets with each leg.

LYING HAMSTRING STRETCH

Targets: Hamstrings, Gastrocnemius

Lie on the floor and grab the back of your left thigh. Keeping your left leg straight, raise it as high as you can without bending your left knee until you feel the stretch in your hamstring and/or calf. Hold for 4–5 deep breaths, or 20–30 seconds. Do 2 sets with each leg.

TRAINER'S TIP

If you're having trouble hanging on to your leg while keeping your back flat, wrap a towel around your thigh or the ball of your foot for leverage. If you can't keep your raised leg straight, try bending the opposite knee.

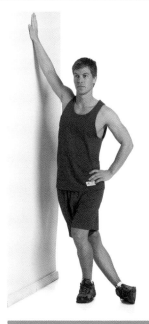

ILIOTIBIAL BAND STRETCH

Targets: Iliotibial Band

Stand with your right side facing a wall; hold the wall with your right hand for support. Keeping your right knee straight, cross your left leg over the right and slowly lean to your left. Gently move your right hip towards the wall until you feel a stretch on the outside of your right hip. Hold 4–5 deep breaths, or 20–30 seconds. Do 2 sets for each side.

LEG RAISE WITH ROTATION, POSITION A

Targets: Quadriceps (especially the Vastus Medialis Oblique), Hip Flexor, Groin

1 Lying flat on your back, bend your left knee and extend your right leg. Turn your right foot slightly outwards.

2 Tighten the muscle at the top of your thigh and slowly raise your right leg until it's almost parallel to your left knee. Hold for 1–2 seconds and slowly lower your right leg to the starting position. Do 20 reps with each leg.

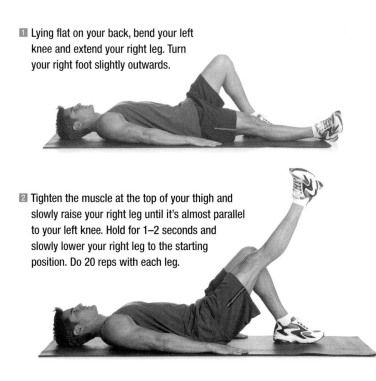

LEG RAISE WITH ROTATION, POSITION B

Targets: Quadriceps (especially the Vastus Medialis Oblique), Hip Flexor, Groin

Start as you did for Position A. Now, sit up slightly and lean back on your forearms and elbows. Tighten the muscle at the top of your thigh and slowly raise your right leg until it's almost parallel to your left knee. Hold for 1–2 seconds and slowly lower your right leg back down to the starting position. Do 20 reps with each leg.

LEG RAISE WITH ROTATION, POSITION C

Targets: Quadriceps (especially the Vastus Medialis Oblique), Hip Flexor, Groin

Again, start as you did for Position A. This time sit up even further and lean back on your hands. Tighten the muscle at the top of your thigh and slowly raise your right leg until it's almost parallel to your left knee. Hold for 1–2 seconds and slowly lower your right leg to the starting position. Do 20 reps with each leg.

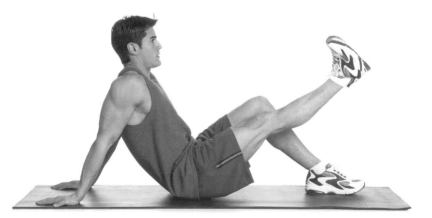

WALL SLIDE

Targets: Buttocks, Hamstrings, Abdominals, Core

Stand with your legs shoulder-width apart and position a Swiss ball between your back and a wall. Place a squeezing block or ball between your knees. With your back straight and your hands on your hips, slowly slide down the wall until your knees bend to about 80–90 degrees. Hold for 10 seconds, then return to the starting position. Do 2 sets of 10 reps.

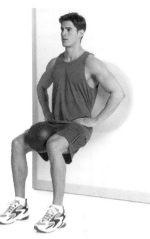

LEG PRESS WITH BALL SQUEEZE

Targets: Inner and Outer Quadriceps, Buttocks, Hamstrings

1 Lie on a leg press machine with your feet on the platform and position a small ball between your knees.

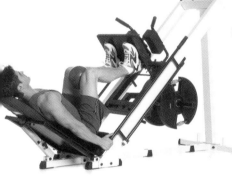

2 Gently squeeze the ball and press the platform upwards until your legs are straight, but not locked. Slowly return to the starting position. Do 15 reps using medium weights followed by 12–15 reps using medium-to-heavy weights.

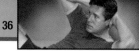

LEG CURL

Targets: Hamstrings

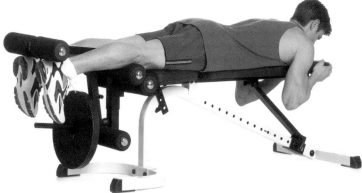

1 Lie on your stomach on a leg curl machine with your legs straight and your heels under the pads.

2 Bring your heels up so your knees are bent to 90 degrees. Slowly return to the starting position. Do 15 reps using a medium weight followed by 12–15 reps using a medium-to-heavy weight.

TRAINER'S TIP

If you have a meniscal injury (see page 26) you may not be able to bend your knees to 90 degrees without pain. Do the curl with your knees bent to 70–80 degrees, or continue to decrease the range of motion until you can do the curl without pain.

PARTIAL QUADRICEPS EXTENSION

Targets: Quadriceps (emphasis on the Vastus Medialis Oblique)

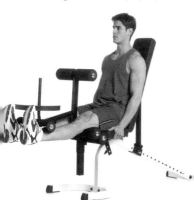

1. Before you begin, set the leg press machine so that your lower legs are at 45 degrees in the starting position. Then, sit in the chair, hook your shins behind the pads and lift your legs to zero degrees, keeping your toes flexed.

2. Slowly lower your legs to the 45-degree starting position. Do 15 reps using a medium weight followed by 12–15 reps using a medium-to-heavy weight.

3. Do 2 final single-leg sets to fatigue, one with each leg, using a medium weight (not pictured).

ONE-FOOT BALANCE

Targets: Foot, Ankle, Hip, Core

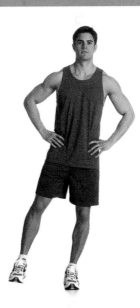

Stand with your legs shoulder-width apart and look straight ahead at a fixed spot. With your arms on your hips, balance on your left leg for 30 seconds. Do 3–4 reps with each leg.

TRAINER'S TIP

If you have an injury, practise balancing on your non-injured leg. Extend your arms out to your sides at shoulder level if you're having trouble keeping your balance for 30 seconds.

STEP UPS AND DOWNS

Targets: Inner and Outer Quadriceps (emphasis on the Vastus Medialis Oblique)

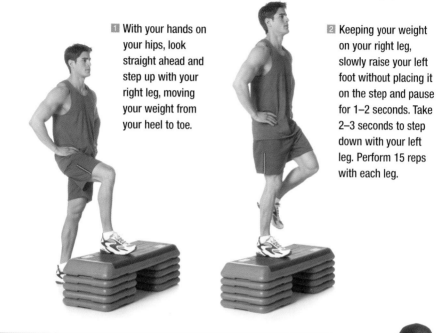

1 With your hands on your hips, look straight ahead and step up with your right leg, moving your weight from your heel to toe.

2 Keeping your weight on your right leg, slowly raise your left foot without placing it on the step and pause for 1–2 seconds. Take 2–3 seconds to step down with your left leg. Perform 15 reps with each leg.

PARTIAL SQUAT WITH OVERHEAD PRESS

Targets: Foot, Ankle, Gastrocnemius, Quadriceps, Buttocks, Core

1 Stand with your feet hip-width apart holding a medium-weight medicine ball at chest level. Squat slightly and turn your toes outwards.

2 Rise up on the balls of your feet and simultaneously press the ball over your head. Hold the position for 3 seconds, then slowly lower your heels to the ground. Do 2 sets of 15 reps.

TRAINER'S TIP

If you have a shoulder or neck injury, avoid pressing the ball overhead.

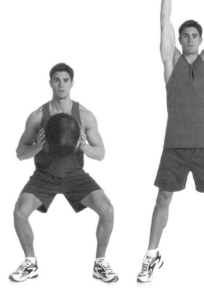

Thigh, Hip and Pelvis Injuries

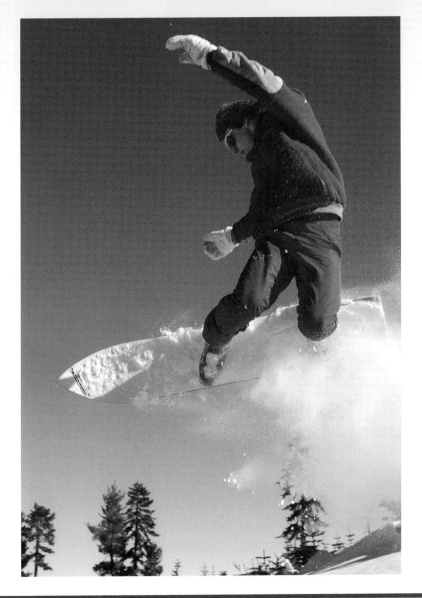

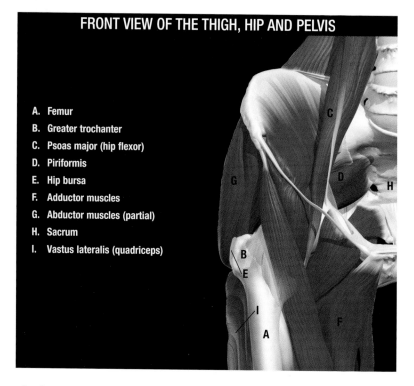

FRONT VIEW OF THE THIGH, HIP AND PELVIS

A. Femur
B. Greater trochanter
C. Psoas major (hip flexor)
D. Piriformis
E. Hip bursa
F. Adductor muscles
G. Abductor muscles (partial)
H. Sacrum
I. Vastus lateralis (quadriceps)

Thigh muscles are a runner's engine. They need strength to power you through a workout and flexibility to help you dig deep and cross the finish line. Most guys are content to build their quadriceps and stretch their hamstrings, but if that's your entire workout, you're going only halfway. Strengthen and stretch all the muscles of your thighs. Keep this area of your body conditioned and you'll avoid a host of problems.

STRESS FRACTURE OF THE FEMUR

How it feels

This injury mimics a groin strain, causing pain along the inside of the leg that can be severe enough to cause a limp. Unlike a strain, the pain comes on gradually.

How it happened

Over-training has caused a hairline fracture in your femur, which is the bone that connects your hip to your knee. This often occurs in endurance sports such as running, when the hip and thigh muscles fatigue and are unable to absorb shock.

How to treat it

The fracture may be too small to show up on an X-ray, so you may need to have an MRI – a test that provides computer-generated images of the body – to confirm the diagnosis. If left untreated, a stress fracture of the femur can progress to a full fracture and require surgery.

How to prevent it

Gradually increase your training distance or speed over time.

HIP BURSITIS
How it feels

You feel pain on the outside of your hip, most noticeably when climbing stairs, walking uphill or downhill, or moving your thigh. It may also hurt to lie on the injured side.

How it happened

Your body comes equipped with its own hip pads – sacs of fluid called bursae – that cover the bones high on the outer side of each thigh. These sacs protect the hip bones from the constant friction of the muscles and tendons moving around it.

If you punish the muscles in and around your hips by over-training – adding too much distance too quickly to your cycling or running routine – you can irritate the bursae, which then swell. A related injury is

tendinitis where your gluteal muscles attach to the outside of the hip. Inflammation of this tendon can also irritate the bursa.

How to treat it

To reduce swelling, ice the area and take non-steroidal pain medication. For severe pain and swelling, you may need a cortisone injection to speed healing. Do the stretches on pages 45–48 to develop flexibility in your hip flexors and thigh muscles. This can help increase your stride length when jogging and can also improve the efficiency of lateral movements in tennis and football.

How to prevent it

Develop the hip and thigh muscles around the area of your injury with the exercises on pages 47–52.

GROIN STRAIN
How it feels

Sudden pain and swelling along the inside of one thigh that may be bad enough to cause a limp.

How it happened

You've stretched or torn the adductor muscles – the ones running along the inner thigh, attached to the pelvis – that help bring your legs together. A sudden lunge can stretch or tear these muscles.

How to treat it

Use ice, non-steroidal pain medication and crutches (if necessary). Also, be aware that you may not have a simple groin strain. If you were playing a contact sport that requires a lot of stopping and starting, notably football or rugby, you may have torn the tendon that attaches the abductor to your pelvis.

Persistent pain high in the groin and lower abdomen that fails rehabilitation may be a Gilmore's Groin, a kind of hernia. The injury develops over time and often resists healing. If the pain is persistent, you may need surgery to close the hernia and to tighten the floor of the pelvis.

Another related injury is osteitis pubis, inflammation at the point where the pubic bones come together in front of the pelvis. It's an injury common to distance runners (and women who have just given birth). The best treatment is rest.

How to prevent it

Warm up your leg muscles with five to ten minutes of cycling or jogging before you head to the gym or play your sport. After your warm-up, do all of the flexibility exercises on pages 45–47. Try to hold each stretch for as long as you comfortably can, without bouncing or pushing to the point where you feel pain.

QUADRICEPS STRAIN

How it feels

There's a sudden pull or pop at the front of your thigh. The sharp pain gives way to a burning and swelling in the quad muscles. It's difficult to walk, to lift your knee or even to bend your leg.

How it happened

You slipped, kicked or lunged suddenly and strained this thick group of muscles. The quadriceps connect your knee to your hip and help you with a host of movements, including running, kicking and rising from a seated position. Tears in these muscles tend to occur in the middle of the thigh, but they can also happen in the upper and lower sections.

How to treat it

Use RICE (see page 8) to treat the injury. Be sure to do a lot of stretching (especially the Quad Stretch on page 31) during rehabilitation to keep the muscles flexible.

How to prevent it

Keep your quadriceps strong so they can absorb the impact of sudden movements without pulling or tearing. Warm up with five to ten minutes of low-impact aerobic exercise, stretch, and do the strengthening exercises on pages 47–52.

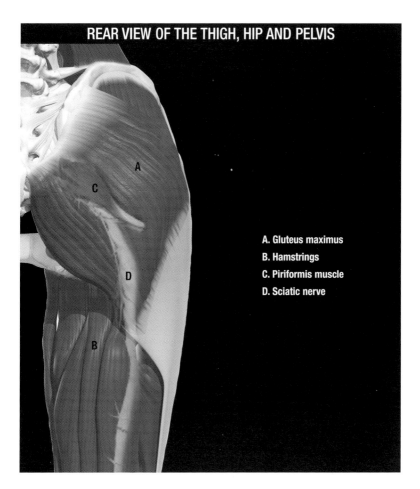

REAR VIEW OF THE THIGH, HIP AND PELVIS

A. Gluteus maximus
B. Hamstrings
C. Piriformis muscle
D. Sciatic nerve

QUADRICEPS CONTUSION

How it feels

There's pain and swelling at the point of impact, followed by bruising. You can't move your knee very much.

How it happened

You sustained a direct blow to the front of your thigh from a ball, a bat or even someone's helmet. Although a

quadriceps contusion (also known as a corked thigh) is usually a contact sport injury, a nasty fall in a sport such as skiing can also be a culprit.

How to treat it

Ice the injury and wrap the muscle to reduce the swelling. Keep the knee bent for as long as possible for the first twenty-four hours so that the leg doesn't stiffen and become almost impossible to bend. If this happens, rehabilitation becomes more difficult. Also keep in mind that as a muscle heals, calcium deposits can form as a kind of scar tissue in the injured area. In this case, your quadriceps won't be able to lift your knee normally and the result will be a temporary limp. To keep this from happening, continually ice and bend your knee. Non-steroidal pain medication also helps prevent calcium deposits.

How to prevent it

If you play any kind of contact sport, make sure you wear protective padding around your thighs.

HAMSTRING STRAIN

How it feels

There is a sudden pull or tearing in your hamstring muscles, maybe even a pop, followed by pain and burning along the back of your thigh. You'll have a hard time walking or putting weight on the injured leg and the muscles will begin to swell. After a couple of days, the area around your injury may bruise.

How it happened

Your hamstrings are a group of muscles at the back of each thigh that allow you to push off, leap, run and bend your leg. Any movement, such

as a jump or a long stride, which suddenly lengthens one of these muscles can tear it. This usually happens in the middle of the muscle, but may occur at either end.

How to treat it

Don't try to walk on it; that will only aggravate the injury. Ice the area around the strain immediately and wrap the muscle in an elastic bandage to control the swelling. You probably don't need to go to hospital unless the pain is excruciating and you're unable to stand. In that case, the muscle may be completely torn and you will need to consult a doctor.

In most cases, the best treatment is rest. The key is to stay off the leg while it heals, which may mean using crutches. It may take a week to a month for you to fully recover from a minor pull; longer if your hamstrings are torn. Be sure your injury has healed completely before hitting the court or the treadmill again to avoid re-injuring the muscle.

How to prevent it

Make sure to warm up thoroughly before your game or workout and don't forget to stretch afterwards. Use the Seated and Lying Hamstring Stretches on page 32. Keep your leg muscles strong and supple with the workout beginning on page 45.

Thigh, Hip and Pelvis Workout

Whether you're recovering from a groin strain or looking for ways to keep your arthritic hip healthy, the following exercises will help you regain and maintain strength, flexibility and range of motion in the hip, pelvis and thigh. Small, precise movements go a long way when training these muscles, so focus on doing each exercise exactly as it is described. If you need to brush up on workout basics, flip to the introduction and re-read the sections on effective warm-up routines and developing a balanced training regime. Finally, review the injury descriptions on pages 40–44 to see whether the following exercises are appropriate for your condition. Consult your doctor if you have additional concerns about physical limitations that may be related to your injury.

SEATED GROIN STRETCH
Targets: Groin, Inner Hamstrings

In a seated position, bring the soles of your feet together in front of you and slowly pull your feet in towards your groin. Keeping your back straight, lean slightly forwards and grab your ankles, placing your elbows on your thighs. Push your thighs down with your elbows until you feel the stretch in your groin. Hold for 4–5 deep breaths, or 20–30 seconds. Do 2 sets.

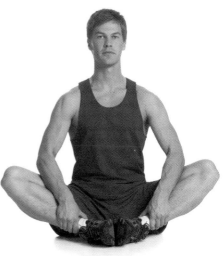

STANDING GROIN STRETCH

Targets: Groin, Inner Hamstrings

Stand with your feet shoulder-width apart and your hands together in front of your chest. Take a big step to the right, as far as you comfortably can. Keeping your right leg straight, lean towards the left by slightly bending your left knee until you feel the stretch in your right inner thigh and/or inner hamstring. Hold for 4–5 deep breaths, or 20–30 seconds.
Do 2 sets with each leg.

HIP FLEXOR-QUAD STRETCH

Targets: Hip Flexors, Quadriceps

Bend down onto your left knee with your right foot forward and your right knee bent to 90 degrees (similar to a lunge position). Lean back slightly and gently pull your ankle up to bend your knee. With your back straight, lean forwards until you feel a stretch in the top of your left thigh and in the front of your left hip. Hold for 4–5 deep breaths, or 20–30 seconds.
Do 2 sets with each leg.

PIRIFORMIS STRETCH

Targets: Piriformis, Iliotibial Band

Lie on your back, with your left ankle crossed over your right knee. Grab your right thigh with both hands and pull your right leg up until you feel a deep stretch in your left buttock. Hold for 4–5 deep breaths, or 20–30 seconds. Do 2 sets with each leg.

LEG RAISE WITH ROTATION, POSITION A

Targets: Quadriceps (especially the Vastus Medialis Oblique), Hip Flexor, Groin

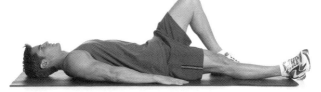

1 Lying flat on your back, bend your left knee and extend your right leg. Turn your right foot slightly outwards.

2 Tighten the muscle at the top of your thigh and slowly raise your right leg until it's almost parallel to your left knee. Hold for 1–2 seconds and slowly lower your right leg to the starting position. Do 20 reps with each leg.

LEG RAISE WITH ROTATION, POSITION B

Targets: Quadriceps (especially the Vastus Medialis Oblique), Hip Flexor, Groin

Start as you did for Position A. Now, sit up slightly and lean back on your forearms and elbows. Tighten the muscle at the top of your thigh and slowly raise your right leg until it's almost parallel to your left knee. Hold for 1–2 seconds and slowly lower your right leg to the starting position. Do 20 reps with each leg.

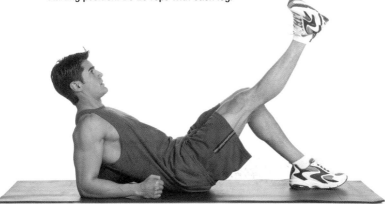

LEG RAISE WITH ROTATION, POSITION C

Targets: Quadriceps (especially the Vastus Medialis Oblique), Hip Flexor, Groin

Again, start as you did for Position A. This time sit up even further and lean back on your hands. Tighten the muscle at the top of your thigh and slowly raise your right leg until it's almost parallel to your left knee. Hold for 1–2 seconds and slowly lower your right leg to the starting position. Do 20 reps with each leg.

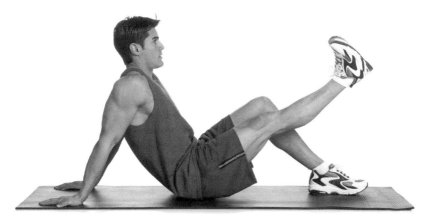

HIP ABDUCTION

Targets: Hip Abductors

1 Lie on your left side with your legs extended, using your left forearm for support.

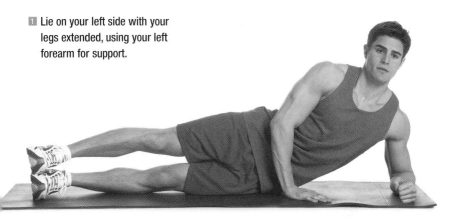

2 Keeping the bottom of your left hip touching the floor, slowly raise your right leg. Hold for 1–2 seconds, then slowly lower your leg to the starting position. Do 2 sets of 15 reps with each leg.

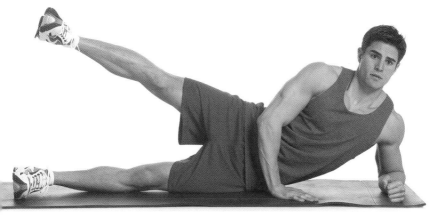

TRAINER'S TIP

Keep both legs straight throughout the exercise, and don't let your body tip forwards or backwards.

HIP ABDUCTION WITH ROTATION

Targets: Hip Flexors, Buttocks, Hamstrings, Hip Abductors

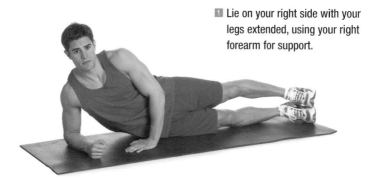

1 Lie on your right side with your legs extended, using your right forearm for support.

2 Keeping the bottom of your right hip touching the floor, raise your left leg towards your head and pause for 1 second.

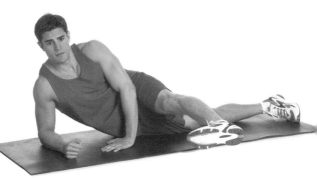

3 Slowly raise your left leg towards the ceiling, as high as you comfortably can without falling backwards. Hold for 1–2 seconds, then slowly return to the starting position. Do 1 set of 15 reps with each leg.

HIP EXTENSION

Targets: Buttocks, Hamstrings, Lower Back

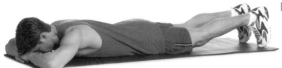

1 Lie on your stomach with your legs extended and your toes on the floor.

2 With your hips touching the floor and your knees a few centimetres off the floor, raise your left leg. (If you feel any lower back pain when you do this, you may be raising your leg too high.) Hold for 1–2 seconds and slowly return to the starting position. Do 2 sets of 15 reps with each leg.

BENT KNEE LIFT

Targets: Buttocks, Hamstrings, Lower Back

1 Lie on your stomach with your right leg extended and the toes of your foot on the floor. Bend your left knee to 90 degrees.

2 Slowly raise your left leg, keeping your left knee bent and your right knee off of the floor. Hold for 1–2 seconds and slowly return to the starting position. Do 2 sets of 15 reps with each leg.

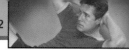

STANDING INNER THIGH SQUEEZE

Targets: Inner Thigh, Groin

TRAINER'S TIP

Do not do this exercise if you have an MCL injury (see page 28).

■ At a cable column, securely attach an ankle cuff to your right ankle. Take a step away from the pulley and stand with your hands on your hips and your feet shoulder-width apart.

■ Standing on your left leg, slowly pull your right leg towards your left. Hold 1–2 seconds, then slowly return to the starting position. Do 2 sets of 15 reps using a medium weight.

Back and Neck Conditions

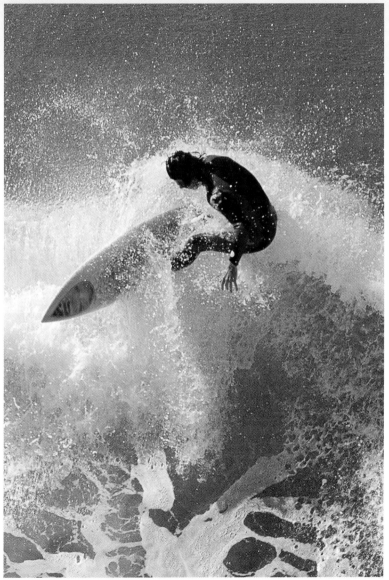

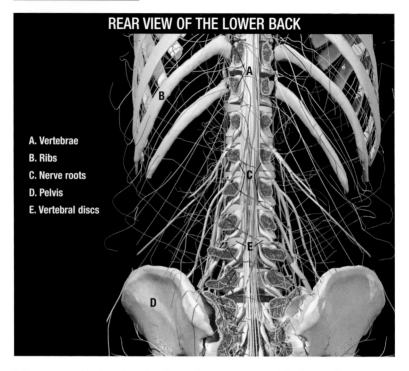

REAR VIEW OF THE LOWER BACK

A. Vertebrae
B. Ribs
C. Nerve roots
D. Pelvis
E. Vertebral discs

Many people develop back problems over a lifetime of gruelling workouts and punishing contact sports. The irony is that the back can withstand abuse until one day you bend over to tie your shoelaces and find that your luck has run out. Improve your chances of staying injury-free by bending at the knees to lift heavy objects and by strengthening your core, abs and lower back. Stretch your back and core muscles regularly, especially before you work out or play your game.

LOWER-BACK PAIN

How it feels

Your lower spine and the muscles that surround it ache. The pain may be worse in the morning or evening and after sitting or driving a car for any length of time. You may also feel pain after working out.

How it happened

Continually stressing the back muscles with poor posture or mechanics will cause injury over time. You can also tear muscles or rupture discs by lifting something incorrectly or bending in an unnatural way. If you tend to work out without warming up and stretching, your back muscles will become tight and prone to injury.

How to treat it

Back pain is the most common medical complaint amongst men aged 30 to 50. Use ice or heat to control the pain and rest the muscles in your back as often as you can. That means getting up from your desk frequently to walk around. Break up long drives, train and bus journeys, or flights by doing the same. Simple stretches such as the Lower-Back Stretch (page 60) can improve flexibility. Strengthen your abdominals and core muscles with the exercises on pages 61–66 to help distribute pressure evenly along your spine.

In the long term, learn new ways to bend and pick up objects so that you don't aggravate your injury. For example, avoid bending over at the waist to lift objects out of the boot of your car. Instead, put your foot up on the bumper, keep your spine stable and bend at your knees as you lift.

How to prevent it

There is no one, simple solution. Incorporate good posture into all your activities. Improve flexibility in your back with the stretches on pages 60–61 and develop your back and core muscles with the strengthening exercises on pages 61–66.

STRESS FRACTURE OF THE LOWER BACK

How it feels

A stress fracture often feels a lot like lower-back pain and can also include sudden spasms of pain.

How it happened

You have injured the vertebrae in your lower back (the knobs you feel along your lower spine) from repetitive motion. Twisting movements or back bends stress the vertebrae and can cause them to break down over time. Eventually, you can develop a stress fracture. There may also be a genetic component at work, so your training methods or choice of sport may not be entirely to blame.

How to treat it

This injury especially hurts when you arch your back, so you'll need to give up the activity that caused the fracture until you can play without pain. In the meantime, ice and anti-inflammatory medication can alleviate some of the pain. You could also consider wearing a brace to prevent further damage. Have some physiotherapy to help strengthen and stabilize the muscles around the injured area. A stress fracture of the lower back will usually sideline you for two to three months and in some cases, can do so for up to a year.

How to prevent it

Begin with the hamstring stretches on page 32. Then, do the crunches on pages 62–63 to strengthen your core. Limit repetitive extensions and rotations (although this is not easy if your sport demands these motions).

HERNIATED DISK

How it feels

With this injury, also known as a ruptured disk, you may feel a sharp pain in one area of the spine that can come on gradually or suddenly. You may feel a jolt of pain when you sit, bend or sneeze. Along with the back pain, you might feel pain, tingling or numbness in one of your legs, a condition called sciatica. The muscles around your spine may seize, making it impossible to stand straight. If you can stand, you may lean to one side. This is your body's way of making itself as comfortable as possible. If the damaged disk is in your neck, you might feel extreme pain while trying to straighten it. You may even feel pain, tingling and numbness in one of your arms.

How it happened

In the space between each vertebra is a disk that works as a shock absorber. If this disk ruptures, the centre bulges out and irritates the nerves around the spine. In some cases, a disk can rupture on its own without much stress.

How to treat it

Control the pain with ice, heat or pain medication. A back or neck brace will help immobilize the area, which will also ease the pain. Your doctor may order an MRI to confirm the diagnosis. Afterwards, you will probably need physiotherapy to strengthen the muscles around the injured area, and to teach you how to bend and lift properly.

How to prevent it

Incorporate all of the stretches and strengthening exercises on pages 59–66 into your workout regime.

WHIPLASH

How it feels

At first, there may be no pain. But slowly, over the course of a day or two, the neck muscles will become sore and stiff. Eventually, you may be unable to move your neck. The pain may extend between your shoulder blades or out onto your shoulders. You may develop a headache.

How it happened

Your neck was forced forwards or backwards into an unnatural position, causing tearing or pulling in several of the muscles that help hold

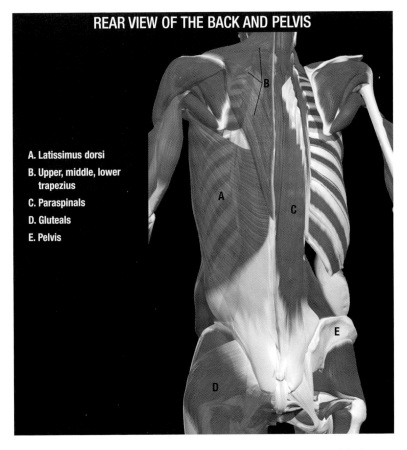

REAR VIEW OF THE BACK AND PELVIS

A. Latissimus dorsi
B. Upper, middle, lower
   trapezius
C. Paraspinals
D. Gluteals
E. Pelvis

your head upright. Whiplash can also mimic an overuse injury caused by bad posture in a sport. A cyclist who rides too far too quickly may suffer whiplash-like symptoms.

How to treat it

Take a non-steroidal, anti-inflammatory medication or over-the-counter painkiller. You may need to wear a cervical collar – a soft, padded collar that holds the neck in a fixed position. These are an effective way to immobilize the neck and help prevent spasms. Your doctor may give you a muscle relaxant to help ease the pain and spasms.

How to prevent it

Strengthen your neck muscles and develop your range of motion with the exercises on pages 59–60. Improve your posture in all your daily activities. At work, use a headset if you spend a lot of time on the phone. Also try to sit with your feet flat on the floor and your knees even with, or lower than, your hips, when working at your computer. Practise the following range of motion moves:

1. Touch your chin to your chest.
2. Tilt your head back and look up.
3. Turn your head from side to side so your chin is almost in line with your shoulder.
4. Tilt your head to one side, so that your ear almost touches your shoulder; repeat on the other side.

MID-BACK STRAIN
How it feels
You feel pain and spasms in the middle of your back. You may be able to pinpoint one spot in the muscle that is tender and swollen.

How it happened
This injury is common amongst shot-putters and wind surfers with bad form. More likely, you were lifting too much weight on an incline press and arched one hip to help finish the rep. In either case, you combined twisting and pushing motions in an unnatural way. This strained the muscles that run along the middle of your spine.

How to treat it
Use ice, non-steroidal pain medication and rest until the pain is gone. Avoid twisting motions as you heal.

How to prevent it
Pay close attention to your form when lifting or doing weight-bearing exercises. It's better to lift less weight and lift it correctly than to show off and hurt yourself. Repeatedly injuring your mid-back muscles can lead to arthritis later in life.

STINGER
How it feels
There's a sudden loss of sensation in one arm for a few minutes, or tingling as if the nerve has gone to sleep. In some cases, you may feel a surge of pain like an electrical charge in the nerve running down the arm.

How it happened
Your head snapped suddenly sideways, stretching the nerves that travel from your neck to your arm.

How to treat it
Stay out of the game until feeling returns to your arm, you regain your strength and you can do complete windmills with a full range of motion. This can sometimes take only a few minutes. If you get a stinger on both sides, you'll need an X-ray.

How to prevent it
Perform the flexibility and strengthening exercises in the workouts on pages 59–66 and 72–78.

Back, Neck and Core Workout

Every move you make originates in your core – the muscles in your torso and back that attach to the spine, pelvis and hips. These muscles work to keep your body upright and stable. By strengthening your entire core you not only minimize the risk of lower-back injuries but also condition and define your abdominals. The following workout is a powerful adjunct to any of the other programmes in this book and will help you achieve muscular balance, strength and flexibility in your lower back and abs. After warming up with 5 to 10 minutes of low-impact aerobic exercise, ease into the workout with the neck and lower back stretches. Then, do the back and abdominal exercises on pages 61–66 in the order in which they appear.

SEATED UPPER-TRAP STRETCH

Targets: Upper Trapezius

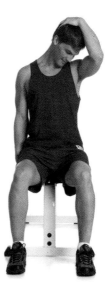

Sit on your right hand with your palm facing up, keeping your shoulders back and your back straight. Turn your head slightly to the left, and look down towards your left knee. To better target your areas of tightness, turn your head slightly more to the left or to the right. With your left hand, gently pull your head in the same direction until you feel the stretch in the right upper trap. Hold for 4–5 deep breaths, or 20–30 seconds. Do 2 sets on each side.

SEATED LEVATOR STRETCH

Targets: Levator

Sit on a bench or chair and rest your right
hand slightly behind your right shoulder.
With your left hand, gently pull your head
to the left until you feel a stretch near
your right shoulder blade. Hold for 4–5
deep breaths, or 20–30 seconds.
Do 2 sets on each side.

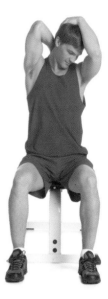

TRAINER'S TIP

The Upper Trapezius and Levator
stretches help relieve tension, stiffness
and pain in the upper back and neck.

LOWER-BACK STRETCH

Targets: Paraspinals, Latissimus Dorsi

1 Start in a kneeling position, facing
a medium-sized Swiss ball. Rest
both hands on the ball and gently
reach forwards while trying to

move your buttocks towards your
heels. Hold for 4–5 deep breaths,
or 20–30 seconds. Do 2 sets.

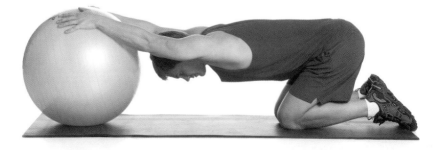

2 Gently reach forwards and turn the ball slightly to the left until you feel a stretch on the right side of your back. Hold for 4–5 deep breaths, or 20–30 seconds. Do 2 sets on each side.

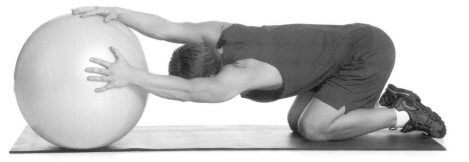

BRIDGE WITH BALL

Targets: Lower Back, Buttocks, Hamstrings

1 Lie on your back with your knees bent and your feet flat on the floor with a light medicine ball between your knees.

2 Keeping your abs tight, gently squeeze the ball and raise your buttocks until your back is straight. Hold for 1–2 seconds and return to the starting position. Do 1 set of 30 reps.

SINGLE LEG BRIDGE

Targets: Lower Back, Buttocks, Hamstrings, Obliques

1 Lie on your back with your knees bent and feet flat on the floor. Straighten your left leg and raise it so it's parallel with your right leg.

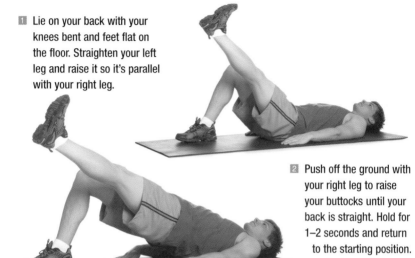

2 Push off the ground with your right leg to raise your buttocks until your back is straight. Hold for 1–2 seconds and return to the starting position. Do 1 set of 20 reps.

MODIFIED CRUNCH, POSITION A

Targets: Abdominals (emphasis on upper abdominals)

1 Lie on your back with your knees bent and your feet flat on the floor. Hold a medium to heavy medicine ball straight above your head.

2 Keeping the medicine ball straight above your head, curl your head and torso towards your knees without using momentum. Hold for 1–2 seconds and slowly return to the starting position. Do 20 reps.

MODIFIED CRUNCH, POSITION B

Targets: Abdominals (emphasis on lower abdominals)

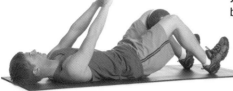

1 Lie on your back with your knees slightly bent and your feet resting on your heels. Place a light medicine ball between your knees and extend your arms over your navel, as pictured.

2 Keeping your arms straight and in line with your navel, squeeze the medicine ball as you slowly raise your knees towards your hands. Hold for 1–2 seconds and return to the starting position. Do 20 reps.

MODIFIED CRUNCH, POSITION C

Targets: Abdominals (emphasis on upper and lower abdominals)

1 Lie on your back with a light medicine ball between your knees and hold a medium to heavy medicine ball straight above your head. Squeeze the ball between your knees and raise your knees towards your hands.

2 Keeping the medicine ball straight above your head, squeeze the ball between your knees as you curl up. Hold for 1–2 seconds and return to the starting position. Do 20 reps.

MODIFIED PLANK

Targets: Pectorals, Deltoids, Abdominals, Lower Back, Buttocks, Core

1 Lie on your stomach with your legs extended behind you and your toes on the floor. Look straight ahead and prop yourself up on your forearms.

2 With your elbows under your shoulders, lift your hips and knees off the mat to straighten your back. Hold for 10 seconds and return to the starting position. Do 10 reps.

MODIFIED PLANK WITH HIP EXTENSION

Targets: Pectorals, Deltoids, Abdominals, Lower Back, Buttocks, Obliques, Core

1 Position your elbows under your shoulders and lift your hips and knees off the mat.

2 While balancing on your forearms and your toes, raise your left leg. (If you feel lower back pain, you may be raising your leg too high.) Hold for 1–2 seconds and return to the starting position. Do 2 sets of 15 reps with each leg.

SIDE LYING PLANK

Targets: Pectorals, Deltoids, Obliques, Lower Back, Core

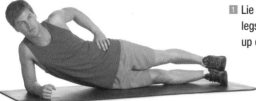

1 Lie on your right side with your legs extended and prop yourself up on your right forearm.

2 With your left arm on your hip, raise your body until your back is straight. Hold for 10 seconds and return to the starting position. Do 10 reps on each side.

SWISS BALL ARM AND LEG EXTENSION

Targets: Paraspinals, Obliques, Buttocks, Hamstrings

1 Lie face-down on a Swiss ball with your palms on the floor and your legs extended behind you, as pictured. Look straight ahead and keep your legs shoulder-width apart for balance.

2 Raise your right arm and left leg simultaneously. Hold for 1–2 seconds and return to the starting position. Do 1 set of 15 reps on each side.

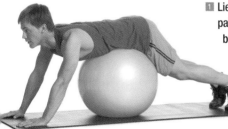

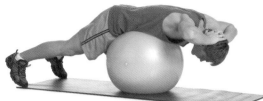

SWISS BALL BACK EXTENSION

Targets: Lower Back, Buttocks

1 Lie face-down on a Swiss ball with your feet slightly more than shoulder-width apart and your toes on the floor. Place your hands behind your head.

2 With your elbows back and in line with your shoulders, raise your upper body by extending your back. Hold for 1–2 seconds and return to the starting position. Do 2 sets of 15 reps.

SWISS BALL BACK EXTENSION WITH ARM EXTENSION

Targets: Lower Back, Buttocks, Lower Trapezius, Paraspinals

1 Lie face-down on a Swiss ball with your feet slightly more than shoulder-width apart and your toes on the floor. Place your hands behind your head, keeping your elbows in line with your shoulders.

2 Raise your upper body by extending your back and straighten your arms. Hold for 1–2 seconds, place your hands behind your head, and slowly return to the starting position. Do 1 set of 20 reps.

Shoulder Injuries

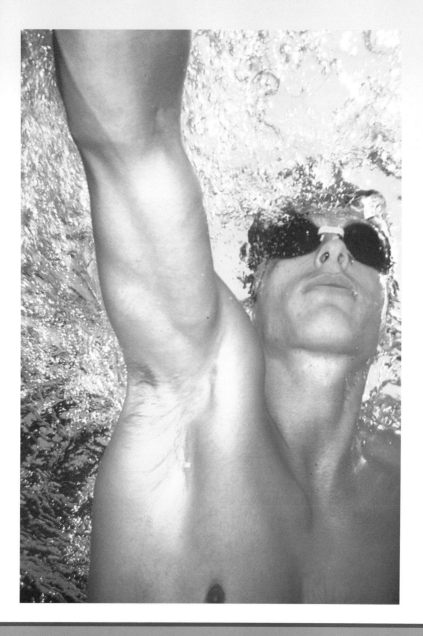

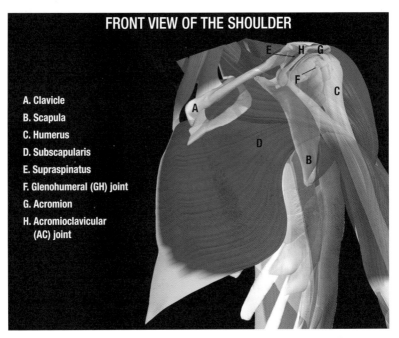

FRONT VIEW OF THE SHOULDER

A. Clavicle
B. Scapula
C. Humerus
D. Subscapularis
E. Supraspinatus
F. Glenohumeral (GH) joint
G. Acromion
H. Acromioclavicular (AC) joint

Your shoulder has – and needs – the widest range of motion of any joint in your body. That's why a strain or break in one of the bones and tissues that make up your shoulder is so debilitating. Every small movement becomes painful. Although most people spend countless hours in the gym working to develop the muscle groups around their shoulders, few spend as much time as they should maintaining the flexibility of their shoulders. Do this, and you may be able to avoid some of these more common shoulder injuries.

SHOULDER DISLOCATION
How it feels

It feels like your shoulder has pulled itself apart, which it has. In a partial dislocation, the pain is sharpest while the joint is out of place and then subsides to a vicious ache after it pops back in. Your arm may feel weak, or even numb, afterwards. In a complete dislocation, the pain is unbearable and you won't be able to move your arm at all. You will also be able to see and feel the ball joint of your upper arm sticking up unnaturally either from in front of or behind your shoulder.

How it happened

The ligaments that normally hold the ball joint of your upper arm in place have been torn or stretched, allowing the joint to slip out. Some people have naturally loose ligaments, and for them, having a shoulder pop out can be fairly common and not caused by an injury.

How to treat it

If you have suffered a partial dislocation, use ice and non-steroidal pain medication to control the swelling and discomfort. Use both of these for the first few days. If you have a complete dislocation, *do not* try to put the joint back together yourself. *Do not* let your friend try to do it. Tissues swell quickly and only a doctor can set things properly. An amateur is likely to tear more ligaments or even break the arm. Just hold the arm in the most comfortable position – close to your body if the joint is sticking out the back and a little bit away from your body if it's sticking out the front. Use ice packs and anti-inflammatory pain medication to control the swelling. Head to hospital immediately.

How to prevent it

Incorporate shoulder-strengthening exercises, such as Modified Lateral Raises, Modified Forward Raises and V Raises (pages 74–75) into your workouts to help prevent partial and total dislocations. If your shoulder has suffered repeated dislocations, surgery is usually the way to go.

BROKEN COLLARBONE

How it feels

Apart from the pain and swelling, you may be able to feel the break if you run your finger along the outline of the clavicle (also known as the collarbone) – but that's going to cause more pain. Sometimes the bone will actually push through the skin. In this case, you should go straight to hospital, because infection could soon set in.

How it happened

When your shoulder hit the concrete (or another hard surface) the collarbone – the thin bone that runs from your breastbone to your shoulder – snapped like a twig. Perhaps you fell onto your outstretched hand, which can also create enough force to break your collarbone.

How to treat it

Don't move the injured arm. When you get to hospital, you'll have an X-ray taken to assess the extent of the damage. After that, you'll get a special kind of splint, called a 'figure-of-8', which will pin back your shoulders

IDENTIFYING YOUR SHOULDER INJURY

You hit the ground hard and you feel severe pain in your shoulder. What happened? It may be one of two types of shoulder separation.

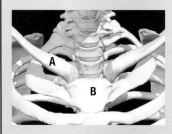

Sternoclavicular Separation (SC Separation) occurs when you tear or sever the ligament that attaches your breastbone to your collarbone, causing pain and swelling near your breastbone. When the ligament tears, it severs the connection between the two bones and may cause the collarbone (A, above) to migrate over or under the sternum (B, above). If it's on top of the sternum, it will simply hurt and swell a lot. A doctor will help move it back into place if needed and splint it so that it heals properly. If the collarbone has moved behind the sternum, it's a medical emergency – you may find yourself in the operating room.

Classic Separation (AC Separation) is a tear in the ligament that connects your collarbone to your shoulder joint. It may be a mild tear in which the shoulder is simply sore, or you may be unable to move your arm. Treat the swollen area with an ice pack for twenty minutes every four hours for the first few days. Take anti-inflammatory medication to reduce the pain and swelling. Your doctor will evaluate the damage and may fit you with a sling to immobilize the arm while the ligaments heal.

slightly (and give you really good posture) or you may just use an ordinary sling. This will help hold the collarbone in place while it heals. Let a doctor decide – by taking another X-ray – when it's time to start playing your sport again. The bone could still be weak and will easily break again.

How to prevent it

If you fall, try to tuck and roll to lessen the impact on your shoulder.

ROTATOR CUFF INJURY
How it feels

The primary symptom is pain when you lift your arm over your head or even above eye level. You may feel a

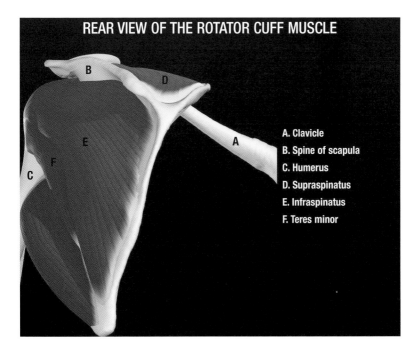

REAR VIEW OF THE ROTATOR CUFF MUSCLE

A. Clavicle
B. Spine of scapula
C. Humerus
D. Supraspinatus
E. Infraspinatus
F. Teres minor

pinching on top or in front of your shoulder. In some cases, you may hear or feel crunching in your shoulder, or as you move your arm or the joint, it may pop a bit. The pain may extend down into your biceps.

How it happened

You injured the tendons in your shoulder joint by doing some kind of repetitive motion, such as swimming or throwing. It's also possible that you fell onto your outstretched arm.

How to treat it

The treatment depends on how serious the injury is. In extreme cases, you may need to have surgery. Usually, however, you'll treat the symptoms and let the shoulder heal on its own. Rest while the pain is severe and use an ice pack at least once a day to reduce swelling. In severe cases, you may need a cortisone injection to reduce the swelling and physiotherapy to restore your range of motion. Once the pain subsides, exercise to strengthen your shoulder muscles.

How to prevent it

Be sure your shoulders are strong enough for the activity you have planned for them. Do the exercises on pages 72–78 and vary your workouts so that you're building the rotator cuff and shoulder blade muscles.

Shoulder Workout

Your shoulders are the most mobile joints in your body. Everyday activities that require you to reach back or overhead and sports like tennis, swimming and skiing all rely on the ability of your shoulder joints to accommodate a wide range of motion. The unfortunate consequence of such versatile mobility is inherent joint instability – the cause of many shoulder injuries. Use the following workout to strengthen your shoulder muscles and develop stability in the supporting joints, tendons and ligaments. Warm up with 5–10 minutes of low-impact cardiovascular exercise. Then, do the stretches to improve flexibility in your shoulder muscles before moving on to the strengthening exercises.

POSTERIOR SHOULDER STRETCH

Targets: Posterior Capsule, Posterior Deltoid, Rotator Cuff

Stand with your feet shoulder-width apart and reach across your body with your left arm. Keeping your left arm straight and your thumb facing the floor, place your right wrist over your left elbow. Gently pull your left arm towards your body until you feel a stretch in the back of your left shoulder. Hold for 4–5 deep breaths, or 20–30 seconds. Do 2 sets with each arm.

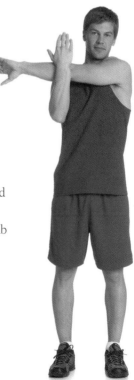

CHEST CORNER STRETCH

Targets: Pectoralis Major, Pectoralis Minor

Stand facing a narrow doorway or a corner and raise your arms so they are parallel to the floor. Bend your elbows to 90 degrees, making an 'L' shape, and rest your forearms on either side of the corner. Take 2 to 3 steps back, and put your feet together. Lean forwards, until you feel a stretch across your chest. Hold for 4–5 deep breaths, or 20–30 seconds. Do 2 sets.

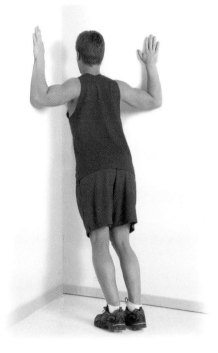

TRICEPS STRETCH

Targets: Triceps, Lower Shoulder Capsule, Rotator Cuff

Standing with your feet shoulder-width apart, reach your right arm over your head and bend your right elbow. With your left arm, grab your right elbow and gently pull back until your feel a stretch in the back of your right arm (triceps region) and/or rear shoulder. Hold for 4–5 deep breaths, or 20–30 seconds. Do 2 sets with each arm.

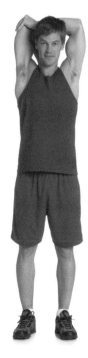

MODIFIED LATERAL RAISES

Targets: Middle Deltoid, Rotator Cuff

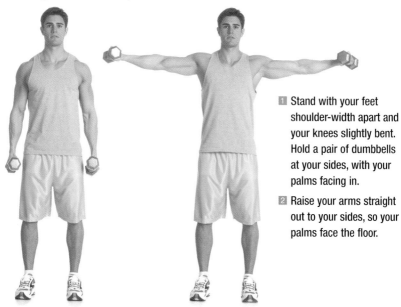

1 Stand with your feet shoulder-width apart and your knees slightly bent. Hold a pair of dumbbells at your sides, with your palms facing in.

2 Raise your arms straight out to your sides, so your palms face the floor.

3 Keeping your left arm straight out to your side at shoulder level, slowly lower your right arm back down to the starting position.

4 Slowly raise your right arm back to shoulder level. Do 2 sets of 8 reps with each arm.

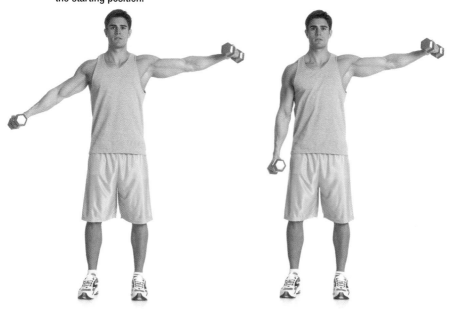

MODIFIED FORWARD RAISES

Targets: Front Deltoid, Pectorals, Rotator Cuff

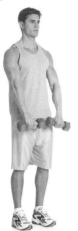
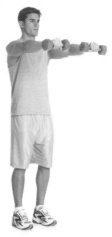
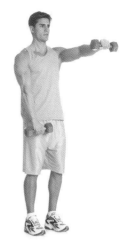

1. Stand with your feet shoulder-width apart and your knees slightly bent. Hold a pair of dumbbells in front of you, with your palms facing your thighs.

2. Raise your arms straight out in front of you, so your palms face the floor.

3. Keeping your left arm straight out in front of you at shoulder level, slowly lower your right arm 90 degrees so it rests in front of your thigh, then raise it back to shoulder level. Do 2 sets of 8 reps with each arm.

'V' RAISES

Targets: Front and Middle Deltoids, Pectorals, Rotator Cuff

1. Stand with your feet shoulder-width apart and your knees slightly bent. Hold the dumb-bells with your palms facing up so the bottom heads nearly touch, as pictured.

2. Slowly raise and lower your arms in a 'V' shape, keeping your arms straight throughout the movement. Do 2 sets of 8 reps with each arm.

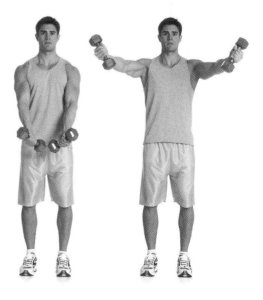

'A', 'T' AND 'Y' RAISES

Targets: Upper, Middle and Lower Trapezius, Rhomboids, Rotator Cuff

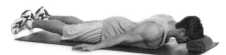

1 Lie face-down on the floor with a towel under your forehead. Start with your legs extended, your toes on the floor, and your arms at your sides, palms down.

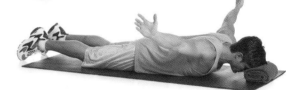

2 Raise your arms as high as you comfortably can while keeping them straight to form an 'A'. Return to the starting position. Do 2 sets of 15 reps.

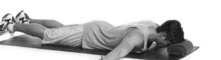

3 Extend your arms out with your palms facing forwards to form a 'T'.

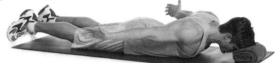

4 Again, raise your arms as high as you comfortably can while keeping them straight. Return to the starting position. Do 2 sets of 15 reps.

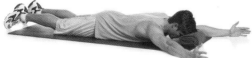

5 Extend your arms out in front of you with your palms facing each other to form a 'Y'.

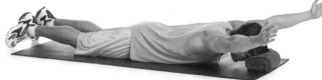

6 Finally, raise your arms as high as you comfortably can. Return to the starting position and complete the last 2 sets of 15 reps.

MODIFIED LAT PULL-DOWN

Targets: Latissimus Dorsi, Posterior Deltoids, Middle Trapezius, Rhomboids

1 Sit on a lat pull-down bench or on a Swiss ball facing a cable column (as shown) with your feet shoulder-width apart and extended slightly forwards. Grasp the bar using a wide overhand grip and lean slightly back from your hips, about 30 degrees, while pushing your chest out.

2 Pull the bar straight back, keeping your elbows wide – away from your body – and your chest out (to prevent any compression of the lower back). Slowly return the bar to the starting position. Do 2 sets of 15 reps.

SIDE LYING EXTERNAL ROTATION

Targets: Rotator Cuff (emphasis on the Supraspinatus and Teres Minor)

1 Lie on your right side, using your right hand to
support your head, and position a small towel
underneath your left elbow to help raise your arm
away from your body and increase blood flow to
the rotator cuff. Hold a dumbbell in your left
hand and bend your elbow 90 degrees, so the
dumbbell is in line with your navel.

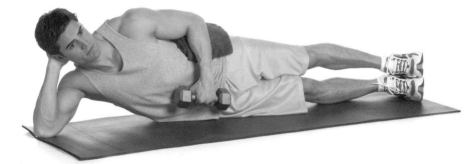

2 Without using momentum, pivot on your left
elbow to raise your arm to hip level. Return to the
starting position. Do 2 sets to fatigue – until you
feel a mild burning sensation in your shoulder
muscles – with each arm.

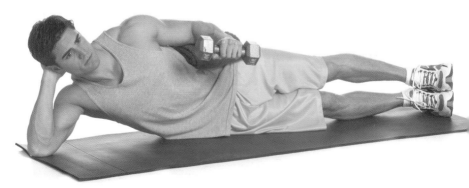

Elbow, Forearm, Wrist and Hand Conditions

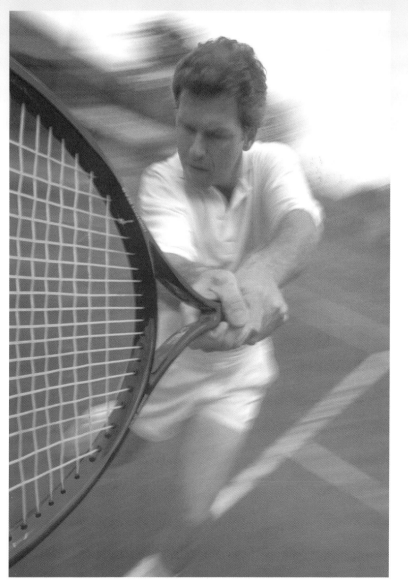

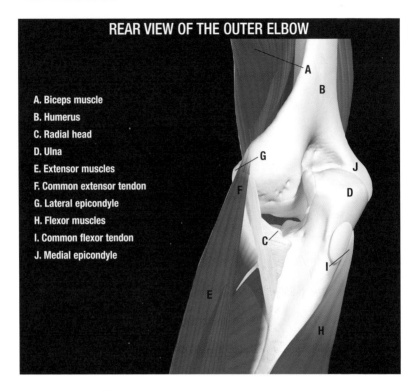

REAR VIEW OF THE OUTER ELBOW

A. Biceps muscle
B. Humerus
C. Radial head
D. Ulna
E. Extensor muscles
F. Common extensor tendon
G. Lateral epicondyle
H. Flexor muscles
I. Common flexor tendon
J. Medial epicondyle

Pain in your elbow is often a sign of weakness in the muscles of your forearm, wrist or hand. In other words, making your elbow do the work that your wrist should be doing can result in torn tendons and swollen nerve tissue that requires many weeks to heal. Athletes who depend on their grip on a handlebar, ball or racquet should pay careful attention to developing strength and flexibility in their hands and wrists. And when the experts tell you to tuck and roll during a fall, they're not kidding. Attempting to break a fall with your arms and hands not only risks sprained or broken wrists and elbows, but also potentially weeks of recovery with the joint immobilized in a brace or cast. If you participate in sports such as skiing or snowboarding, in which falling is part of the fun, practise tucking and rolling to give your elbows, forearms, wrists and hands a rest.

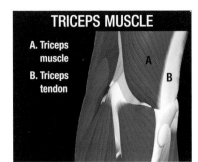

TRICEPS MUSCLE

A. Triceps muscle

B. Triceps tendon

GOLFER'S ELBOW

How it feels

The bone on the inside of your elbow is swollen and painful. It hurts to open or close jars and to play your favourite sports such as golf, softball or tennis.

How it happened

During the downstroke of your golf swing, the club decelerates abruptly as you hit the turf, deep wet sand or a buried root. Or, you frequently play sports that require repetitive swinging or throwing motions. In either case, you've stressed the flexor tendon that attaches the inside of your elbow (medial epicondyle) to your forearm. This causes tiny tears in the flexor tendon over time.

How to treat it

Ice the injury and take non-steroidal, anti-inflammatory medication to treat the immediate symptoms. Try another sport for a few weeks to allow the tendon to heal. In the meantime, improve the range of motion in your wrist and forearm with the stretches on page 91. Strengthen the muscles in your forearm and wrist using the exercises on pages 92–94. It also wouldn't hurt to have a golf pro evaluate your swing.

How to prevent it

Try not to increase your activity level in golf or related sports too suddenly. Add the exercises on pages 92–94 to your workout to strengthen the muscles in your wrists and forearms. Be aware of your pain level as you play, and quit when the tendons in your elbows start to protest.

TENNIS ELBOW

How it feels

The bony bump on the outside of your elbow (lateral epicondyle) is sore and swollen. The pain increases when you pick up things, turn your wrist or shake hands. You may have shooting pain down the length of the extensor tendons.

How it happened

Holding and swinging a racquet or golf club works the tendons of the forearm, especially those that raise and straighten the wrist. If the muscles in your forearms are weak, or if your form is poor, your tendons have to do the majority of the work when swinging. Over time, the tendons suffer small tears. If you hit a tree root hard on your golf swing, you may develop tennis elbow in your non-dominant hand – a similar mechanism of injury as with poor backhand form in tennis. You may also develop tennis elbow if you work out using too much weight, or do too many repetitions with poor form and technique. Sometimes just accidentally hitting your elbow can start the process.

How to treat it

There are many different treatments for tennis elbow. Always begin with the basics: rest, ice packs, anti-inflammatory medicines and massage. If the pain returns and becomes chronic, you may want to think about getting a cortisone injection from your doctor (see page 84), acupuncture, physiotherapy or using a tennis elbow splint. Some doctors feel that one injection of cortisone is worth a month of pain medication. Surgery should only be considered as a last resort.

How to prevent it

Improve flexibility and strengthen your forearm muscles with the stretches and exercises beginning on page 91. Most of all, maintain good form no matter what your sport.

ULNAR NEUROPATHY
How it feels

You feel pain, tingling and numbness in the fourth and fifth fingers of your hand. Although this condition is sometimes called Painful Pinky, the problem actually originates in your elbow. If you tap your funny bone – the area where the ulnar nerve crosses your elbow joint – you will feel that nerve all the way to the tip of your pinky. You may also feel pain and swelling on the inside of your elbow near your funny bone.

How it happened

You took a blow to the inside of your elbow or overextended it. This stretched and irritated the ulnar nerve, which runs along the inside of your elbow to your hand and helps you move and feel your pinky. The tissues around the nerve are swollen and cause pain, tingling or numbness in your pinky.

How to treat it

Take a break from any activity that is causing the injury, which could be gymnastics, martial arts, cycling or racquet sports. Unfortunately, professional athletes who suffer from ulnar neuropathy and fail in rehab usually need surgery. Fortunately, you probably won't. You will need to give up your sport for two weeks to a month

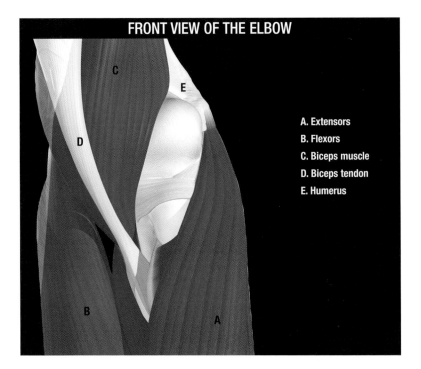

FRONT VIEW OF THE ELBOW

A. Extensors
B. Flexors
C. Biceps muscle
D. Biceps tendon
E. Humerus

while your ulnar nerve heals. You can wear a brace to prevent irritation of the nerve while it mends.

How to prevent it
Pay close attention to your form and avoid putting stress on the inside of the elbow. If you ride a bicycle often, change your grip on the handlebars frequently, or wear padded cycling gloves to absorb vibration.

ELBOW FRACTURE
How it feels
The pain is centred in the bones of the elbow, particularly on the top. You probably find it difficult to twist your wrist from side to side as you would when turning a doorknob. The swelling may be so severe that you can't straighten your arm.

How it happened
The radius – the bone running from your elbow to the thumb side of your wrist – breaks from a fall onto an outstretched arm during a game or after slipping on a wet surface.

How to treat it
You'll need to get an X-ray to find out whether the radius bone is broken – and if it is, how badly. The bone can simply be cracked or it

may be broken in several places. Depending on the severity and location of the fracture, you'll need to wear a splint for several weeks. You won't be able to start rehabilitation exercises until the pain is under control.

How to prevent it

There isn't much you can do to prevent an elbow fracture other than wear elbow pads and try not to fall.

POSTERIOR ELBOW PAIN

How it feels

The back of your elbow hurts, especially when you try to straighten it or lock it out. At times the swelling can be severe; you may be unable to straighten your arm. If you try to throw something, your elbow hurts at the point of release.

How it happened

Forcefully locking out your elbow hundreds of times while throwing a ball can cause swelling in the joint.

How to treat it

A combination of exercise and physiotherapy can quieten the pain. After the inflammation calms down, the pain should, too. Avoid locking out your elbow while you recover.

How to prevent it

Scale back activities that cause pain and strengthen the muscles in your wrists and forearms with the exercises on pages 92–94. Pay attention to your throwing form. Sometimes if you have pain on the inside of your elbow, near the funny bone, you'll over-compensate when you throw.

CORTISONE INJECTIONS

When your doctor tells you that your injury may require an injection of cortisone, here is what he's talking about. Cortisone is a powerful medication that decreases swelling in injured joints and tissues. It is injected directly around swollen ligaments and tendons to begin to shrink the swelling. Reducing the swelling will reduce your pain and can even speed the healing process, getting you back into the game quicker. That's the good news.

The bad news is that it doesn't work right away. In fact, you may experience a cortisone 'flare', in which your pain gets worse about a day after the shot. Then, after several days to a week, you'll notice a significant reduction in pain. In the meantime, you'll need to continue your ice packs, elevation and rest.

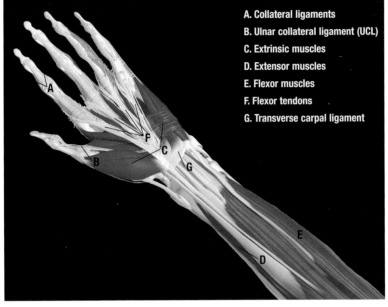

PALM-UP VIEW OF THE HAND, WRIST AND FOREARM (MUSCLES)

A. Collateral ligaments
B. Ulnar collateral ligament (UCL)
C. Extrinsic muscles
D. Extensor muscles
E. Flexor muscles
F. Flexor tendons
G. Transverse carpal ligament

CARPAL TUNNEL SYNDROME

How it feels

You feel pain on the heel of your hand, the fleshy area at the base of your thumb. Or, you feel pain and numbness in the thumb and first three fingers in your hand or even in your forearm. This pain and numbness is worse at night because your wrist tends to flop over while you sleep and increases pressure on the median nerve, which runs from your forearm into your hand through a 'tunnel' in your wrist. This causes the tingling and pain that are the hallmarks of carpal tunnel syndrome. The symptoms may become so severe you have to shake your hands in the morning to restore feeling to the fingers. If this condition is allowed to persist for several months, you may find it difficult to hold objects, and your hands will become more sensitive to cold temperatures.

How it happened

It's not only computer geeks who get carpal tunnel syndrome. Anyone who engages in repetitive activities that require a fixed position of the wrist and forearm for long periods – cyclists, and tennis or racquetball players – can develop the condition. You put pressure on the median nerve by leaning on something for

PALM-UP VIEW OF THE HAND, WRIST AND FOREARM (BONES)

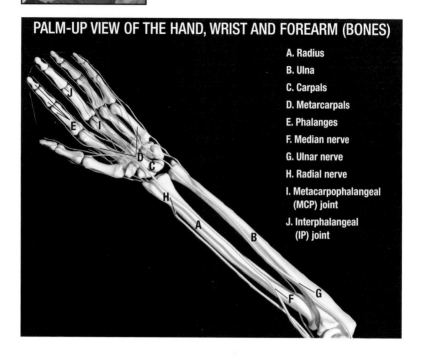

A. Radius

B. Ulna

C. Carpals

D. Metarcarpals

E. Phalanges

F. Median nerve

G. Ulnar nerve

H. Radial nerve

I. Metacarpophalangeal (MCP) joint

J. Interphalangeal (IP) joint

too long, by gripping something too tightly or by performing other repetitive motions such as typing on a keyboard with your wrist in an awkward position. Repeatedly pinching this nerve over many weeks or months causes it to become inflamed. The tissues surrounding the nerve may also be swollen.

How to treat it

First, stop doing whatever you were doing to cause the injury. Second, wear a brace to keep your wrist still at night. If the condition resists treatment, your doctor may inject cortisone into the carpal tunnel area or may even recommend surgery. Your doctor will also tell you to take vitamin B6 or a non-steroidal pain medication to relieve symptoms.

How to prevent it

Avoid the positions that cause symptoms. Adjust your wrist position while working at the computer, change your grip frequently while cycling and, most importantly, address your symptoms early.

SPRAINED FINGER JOINT
How it feels

The finger is swollen and painful. It may also be pointing in an unnatural direction. In this case, the finger might be broken or dislocated.

How it happened

If one of your fingers is jammed, you've injured the tendons and ligaments around the MCP or IP joints. If it's dislocated, the bones have pulled away from the joint.

How to treat it

If your finger is sore, you can usually shake off the pain and continue playing. After the game, ice the finger and restrict its movement by taping it to the next finger. If the pain and stiffness persist for more than forty-eight hours or worsen, have the finger X-rayed. You may have cracked or chipped one of the finger bones.

How to prevent it

The only way to prevent a sprain is to keep the finger out of the line of fire.

WRIST SPRAIN

How it feels

The entire wrist hurts and is difficult to move; the back of the wrist is swollen. The skin may become tender as the swelling increases. You may hear a clicking sound when you try to move the wrist.

How it happened

The bones in your wrist are connected to one another – and to the bones in your hand and your forearm – by a series of ligaments. Any forced movement, such as a fall, a tackle or a blow from a ball can stretch or tear one of these ligaments.

How to treat it

Ice the injury for twenty minutes every four to six hours for a few days. Wrap your wrist in an elastic bandage or wear a brace to immobilize it for a few weeks. Avoid contact sports until you regain full range of motion without pain.

How to prevent it

Wear wrist guards and do your best not to fall on your hands.

ULNAR-COLLATERAL SPRAIN

How it feels

You feel pain centred on the ulna-collateral ligament, the fleshy part of your palm at the base of the thumb.

A BREAK OR A JAM?

It may feel like a sprain or dislocation, but you need to make sure your finger isn't broken. The 'can you move it' test isn't as reliable as an X-ray. Try this instead: make a fist. If one of the fingers seems to point to or even cross the finger next to it, go to hospital. It's probably broken.

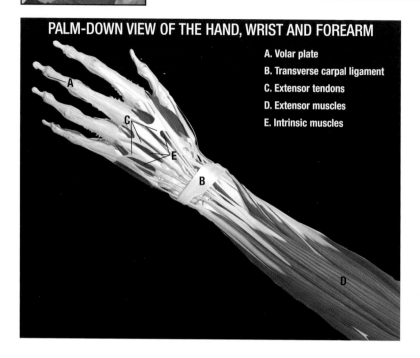

PALM-DOWN VIEW OF THE HAND, WRIST AND FOREARM

A. Volar plate
B. Transverse carpal ligament
C. Extensor tendons
D. Extensor muscles
E. Intrinsic muscles

The area will be swollen and you may experience difficulty moving your thumb or holding objects. In some severe cases, the thumb will feel loose in the joint, as though it's not really attached anymore.

How it happened

Ligaments hold the big knuckle at the base of your thumb together. When you fell, your thumb bent back and the ligament closest to your forefinger tore a bit. In some severe cases, the ligament may have been severed. Skiers frequently suffer from ulnar collateral strain because their thumbs often get tangled in their ski poles as they fall.

How to treat it

Ice the sprained ligament for twenty minutes every four to six hours for the first couple of days to reduce swelling. A non-steroidal, anti-inflammatory medication will also reduce pain and swelling. If the injury is minor, meaning the joint doesn't feel loose, these treatments should be enough. If the injury is more severe, you may need a splint or a cast – some extreme cases may even require surgery.

How to prevent it

Wear gloves with protective plates built in to help keep your thumbs safe during a fall.

EXTENSOR TENDON STRAIN

How it feels

You have sharp pain in the last joint of one of your fingers. The injured finger is bent and cannot be straightened. The tip of the finger is also swollen and tender.

How it happened

The last joint on your finger got jammed, pushing it down towards your palm and past the point where nature intended. The extensor tendon that allows you to straighten that finger has torn away from the bone. It some severe cases, it may have even taken some of the bone with it.

How to treat it

You will need to wear a splint on the injured finger for six to twelve weeks. This will probably heal the injury and allow you to once again straighten your finger. In many cases, you will be left with a slight, yet permanent, bend in the injured joint. Without the splint, there's a chance that the finger will become deformed, so immediate medical attention is important.

How to prevent it

The best way to prevent this injury is to stay alert and use proper form when playing sports like hockey, softball or cricket.

LET YOUR DOCTOR DIAGNOSE

Self-diagnosing a wrist fracture can be tricky business, because symptoms that seem to indicate a break – intense pain and swelling that prevents movement – could actually be caused by a less serious injury. On the other hand, some fractures don't show up immediately – even on X-rays.

For instance, in the case of a thumb-side fracture, your wrist will feel tender and will swell on the thumb side of your wrist. Even after an X-ray, the thumb-side bone (called the scaphoid bone) may not look broken. In that case, the doctor may schedule another X-ray after a week to ten days. Unfortunately, it can take up to three months in a cast to heal because the scaphoid heals slowly.

In other cases, what feels like a wrist fracture could actually be the break of a bone in your forearm – the distal radius.

The lesson? Unless you're absolutely sure your wrist injury is not a fracture, it's a good idea to have a doctor make the diagnosis.

Elbow, Forearm, Wrist and Hand Workout

Common daily activities – housework-related lifting or extended periods typing – can put a lot of pressure on the joints and muscles in your elbows, forearms, wrists and hands. And continually exerting force on these muscles and joints can lead to overuse injuries such as tennis elbow and carpal tunnel syndrome. Because these muscles are small, resistance training with light weights to build overall endurance and stamina – as opposed to size – is key. After warming up with 5 to 10 minutes of low-impact aerobic exercise, use the flexibility exercises to help decrease tension caused by prolonged inflammation associated with posterior elbow pain, tennis and golfer's elbow. Then, do the strengthening exercises in the order they appear below.

Take the time to warm up your muscles with ten to twenty minutes of light jogging and flexibility training before you start the match – this is key to staying injury-free.

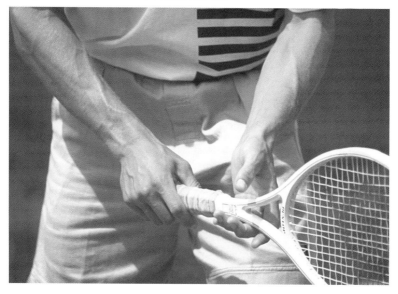

WRIST/HAND FLEXOR STRETCH

Targets: Wrist and Hand Flexors

Stand with your arms straight out in front of you and extend your right wrist, palm out. With your left hand, gently pull your right hand back until you feel the stretch in your right inner forearm. Hold for 5 deep breaths, or 20–30 seconds. Do 2 sets with each hand.

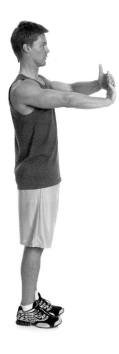

WRIST/HAND EXTENSOR STRETCH

Targets: Wrist and Hand Extensors

Stand with your arms straight out in front of you and point your right thumb towards the floor, so your palm is facing in. With your left hand, gently pull your right hand towards you until you feel the stretch in the top of your right forearm. Hold for 5 deep breaths, or 20–30 seconds. Do 2 sets with each hand.

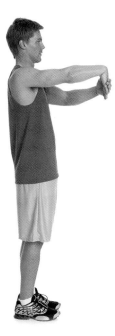

BICEPS CURL

Targets: Biceps, Brachial Radialis

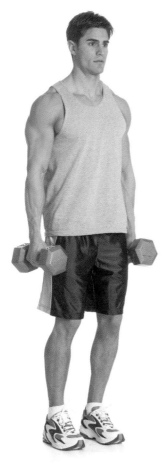

1 Stand with your legs shoulder-width apart and knees slightly bent, holding a pair of dumbbells with your palms facing your thighs.

2 Curl the dumbbells through a ¾ range of motion, turning your palms up towards the ceiling. Return to the starting position. Do 2 sets of 15 reps.

TRAINER'S TIP

Strengthening your biceps muscles, which cross over both the shoulder and elbow joints, helps develop stability in the joints, tendons and ligaments in your elbows.

WRIST ROLLER

Targets: Wrist and Forearm Extensors

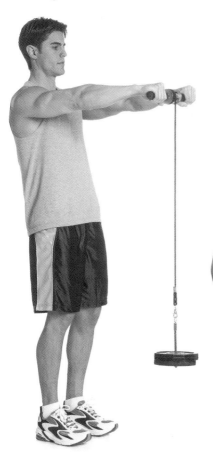

1 Stand with your legs shoulder-width apart and your arms extended straight out in front of you holding an unwound wrist roller (the weight should be near the floor).

2 Keeping your arms parallel to the floor, slowly roll the weight upwards, leading with your right hand. Perform 3 reps leading with your right hand, then do 3 reps leading with your left.

WRIST CURLS

Targets: Wrist and Hand Flexors (palms down), Wrist and Hand Flexors (palms up)

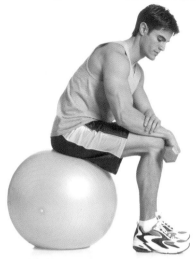

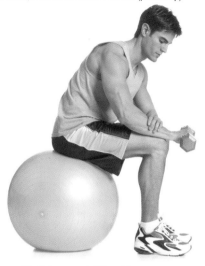

1 Sit on a Swiss ball holding a dumbbell with your right hand palm down, so it hangs in front of your knee.

2 Using your left hand for support, extend your wrist upwards. Do 2 sets of 15 reps with each hand.

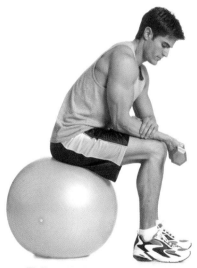

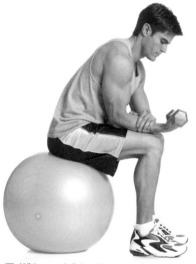

3 To target your wrist and hand flexor muscles, hold the dumbbell in your right hand with your palm up.

4 With your left hand on your forearm, extend your right wrist upwards. Do 2 sets of 15 reps with each hand.

INDEX

ABOUT THE AUTHORS

Dr Brian Halpern, author of *The Knee Crisis Handbook*, is a sports medicine doctor at the Hospital for Special Surgery in New York. He is on the medical staff of the New York Mets baseball team and President of the Foundation of the American Medical Society for Sports Medicine.

Marty Jaramillo, PT, is a sports physiotherapist, athletic trainer and strength and conditioning specialist. A former member of the medical staffs of the New York Knicks basketball team, St John's University and the 1996 Olympic Games, he is Founder & CEO of The I.C.E. Sports Health Group at The Sports Club/LA in New York.

Michelle Seaton, is a medical writer and co-author of *The Cardiac Recovery Handbook*.